Mediterranean Diet Cookbook

2nd Edition

61 Mediterranean Recipes That Keep You Slim & Healthy

by Olivia Rogers

Copyright © 2017 By Olivia Rogers
All rights reserved. No part of this book may be reproduced in any form without permission in writing from the author. No part of this publication may be reproduced or transmitted in any form or by any means, mechanic, electronic, photocopying, recording, by any storage or retrieval system, or transmitted by email without the permission in writing from the author and publisher.
For information regarding permissions write to author at
Olivia@TheMenuAtHome.com
Reviewers may quote brief passages in review.

Please note that credit for the images used in this book go to the respective owners. You can view this at: TheMenuAtHome.com/image-list

Olivia Rogers
TheMenuAtHome.com

Table of Contents

Who is this book for? 6
What will this book teach you? 7
Introduction 8
1. Mediterranean Fresh Sandwich 9
2. Couscous with Orange Juice and Raisins 11
3. Pasta with Shrimp and Tomato Garlic Sauce 13
4. Grilled Tuna Steaks with Tomato Sauce 15
5. Rosemary-Garlic Lamb 17
6. Cooked Lentil with Red Grapes and Mint 20
7. Mediterranean Greek Chicken Vegetable Salad 22
8. Grilled Salmon with Olive Oil and Rosemary 24
9. Grilled Tuna with Olive Dressing 25
10. Sardine and Chickpea Greek Salad 26
11. Spaghetti with Cottage Cheese 28
12. Tangy Chickpeas Salad 29
13. Mediterranean Burger 30
14. Healthy Peanut Salsa 32
15. Plum Tomatoes and Feta Cheese Salsa 33
16. Gluten-Free Corn Salad 34
17. Roasted Bell Peppers and Zucchini Salad 35
18. Plum Tomatoes and Feta Cheese Salsa 36
19. Grilled Chicken Salad 37
20. Garden Fresh Mediterranean Salsa 38
21. Couscous with Cottage Cheese 39
22. Fruit and Cream Mexican Roll 40

23. Black Olives and Corn Mexican Cream Roll _____ 41
24. Assorted Corn Macaroni Salad _____ 42
25. Toasted Quinoa with Tomatoes and Parsley _____ 44
26. Beet and Fennel Salad with Low Fat Dressing _____ 45
27. Mediterranean Fish Stew _____ 47
28. Chopped Lamb with Lettuce _____ 48
29. Spicy Grilled Shrimp _____ 49
30. Healthy Olive Mushroom Salad _____ 50
31. Lemony Grilled Chicken _____ 51
32. Quinoa Salad with Lemon Garlic Dressing _____ 52
33. Quinoa Tabbouleh _____ 54
34. Beet, Blood Orange, Kumquat & Quinoa Salad _____ 56
35. Chickpea Bajane _____ 58
36. Cajun Crab & Quinoa Cakes _____ 60
37. Med Tuna Salad _____ 62
38. Med Chicken Wrap _____ 64
39. Chicken with Mustard, Greens, Olives, and Lemon _____ 66
40. Stuffed Red Peppers _____ 68
41. Med Feta Salad with Pomegranate Dressing _____ 70
42. Orange, Anchovy, & Olive Salad _____ 72
43. Spiced Turkey with Avocado/Grapefruit Relish _____ 74
44. Med Halibut Sandwiches _____ 76
45. Med Salmon _____ 78
46. Med Breakfast Couscous _____ 79
47. Med Basmati Salad _____ 81
48. Artichoke Provencal _____ 83
49. Vegetable and Garlic Calzone _____ 85

50. Tuscan White Bean Stew _____ 87
51. Roasted Cod with Warm Tomato-Olive-Caper Tapenade __ 89
52. Med Grilled Vegetable Tagine _____ 91
53. Barley and Roasted Tomato Risotto _____ 93
54. Braised Kale with Cherry Tomatoes _____ 95
55. Roasted Eggplant and Feta Dip _____ 97
56. Honey and Olive Oil Zucchini Muffins _____ 99
57. Arugula Salad with Cucumber, Feta, and Mint _____ 101
58. Arugula-Pear Salad with Parmesan and Walnuts _____ 103
59. Avocado Gazpacho _____ 105
60. Avocado-Watermelon Salsa _____ 107
61. Black Bean, Edamame, and Wheat Berry Salad _____ 108
Top Fitness Tips of Today! _____ 110
Final Words _____ 111
Disclaimer _____ 113

Who is this book for?

Mediterranean diet enables complete nourishment of a healthy body. It helps to maintain a slim, toned, and healthy physique.

People suffering from obesity are at high risk of cardiovascular diseases. Obesity is the root cause of several diseases such as hyper tension, sleeping disorders and illness of vital organs such as heart, liver and kidneys.

Mediterranean diet is known to minimize the risk of cardiovascular diseases, cancer, Alzheimer's disease and type-2 diabetes. Olive oil is the corner stone of this healthy diet. It is a rich source of healthy fats, vitamin E, phytonutrients and antioxidants.

What will this book teach you?

The book aims to provide healthy and easy to make Mediterranean recipes that help to lose weight and maintain a healthy body.

Delicious burgers, sandwiches, cream rolls and salads can now be prepared with healthy fat substitutes. Most of the recipes are made with fresh vegetables and fruits.

The recipes include healthy salad dressings, low calorie cream rolls and appetizing main course dishes that would satisfy your taste buds without compromising on your heath.

Introduction

This book contains healthy Mediterranean recipes. Fresh vegetables, fruits, olive oil and low-fat ingredients are used to make these recipes nutritious. Olive oil is the vital ingredient used in this diet.

Mediterranean recipes are prepared with olive oil, a healthy source of fat with countless benefits. Olive oil is known to reduce weight, reduce cholesterol levels, and help fight several diseases.

Delicious sandwiches, burgers, salads and other main course dishes can be prepared with healthy fat substitute and healthy salad dressings.

1. Mediterranean Fresh Sandwich

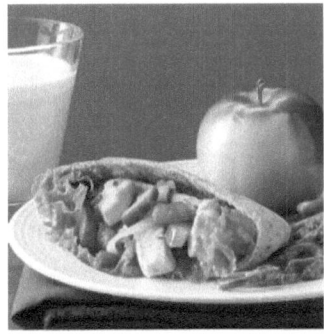

Mediterranean Fresh Sandwich is prepared with fresh vegetables. The sandwich contains cottage cheese, which is a rich source of protein. Olive oil is used for grilling the vegetables, which makes this recipe healthier. The sandwich can be easily prepared and packed within minutes for a lunch or picnic.

Ingredients

- 1 large bread loaf
- 2 tbsp. olive oil
- 1 zucchini sliced into 1/4 inch lengthwise
- 1 eggplant sliced into 1/4 inch lengthwise
- 1 red bell pepper sliced into 1/4 inch lengthwise
- 1/3 cup pesto
- 1/3 cup tapenade
- 1 8 oz. low sodium cottage cheese sliced
- 2 tbsp. of balsamic vinegar
- Salt and pepper as per taste

Method

1. Brush the vegetables with olive oil and grill until they turn soft. Hollow the inside of bread. Spread pesto and tapenade on one side of the bread. Then layer the grilled vegetables and cottage cheese.

2. Drizzle olive oil and balsamic vinegar. Season with salt and pepper. Press the sandwich and wrap tightly with a paper wrap.

3 Reasons Cottage Cheese Helps Reduce Weight

Cottage cheese is a rich source of protein and low in fat content. It also provides the body with the required amount of calcium and Vitamin B.

2. Couscous with Orange Juice and Raisins

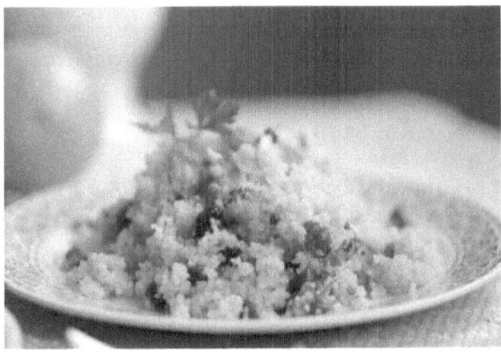

Couscous with orange juice and raisins is a low-calorie dish filled with the goodness of orange juice, raisins and carrots. Slowly stirred couscous with orange juice over medium heat gives this dish a fine texture.

Ingredients

- 1 1/3 cups couscous
- 1/2 cup soaked raisins
- 1 cup orange juice without pulp
- 1 1/3 cups of grated carrots
- 1 tsp cinnamon powder
- 1 tsp olive oil
- Salt and pepper as per taste

Method

1. Heat olive oil in a pan and toast couscous to light brown. Pour in orange juice and 1 cup water. Season with salt and pepper. Bring to a boil and add grated carrots.

2. Cook over low heat stirring in between till the liquid is absorbed. Stir in raisins and cinnamon powder.

3 Reasons to Add Carrots and Oranges to Your Diet

Carrots are regarded as the world's healthiest food. It is a rich source of Vitamin A that helps to improve vision, prevent cancer, and cardiac illness. Oranges promote a healthy heart, lower cholesterol levels, and help fight diseases.

3. Pasta with Shrimp and Tomato Garlic Sauce

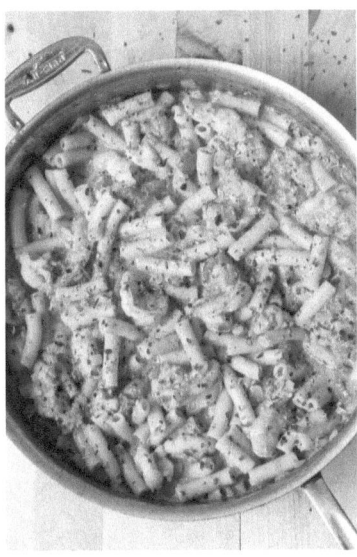

This pasta dish is ready in 20 minutes. Shrimp cooked in a garlic tomato sauce give this dish a new taste. This low-calorie recipe satisfies the taste buds and health equally.

Ingredients

- 1 tsp olive oil
- 1 cup deveined shrimp
- 6 oz. angel hair pasta
- 1 cup diced tomatoes
- 1/2 cup chopped red bell pepper
- 2 tbsp. minced garlic
- Salt and pepper for seasoning
- 5 tbsp. crumbled feta cheese

Method

1. Cook pasta as per package instructions. Heat olive oil in a skillet and sauté tomatoes, bell pepper, and garlic.

2. Now add shrimp, salt, and pepper. Cover and cook until shrimp are done. You can tell when the shrimp are done when their color loses its transparency, and curled into a "c" shape. If it has curled into an "o" shape it is over cooked. Arrange cooked pasta on a platter. Top with shrimp mixture and cheese.

Cooking Tips

Shrimp can be replaced with shredded chicken as well.

4. Grilled Tuna Steaks with Tomato Sauce

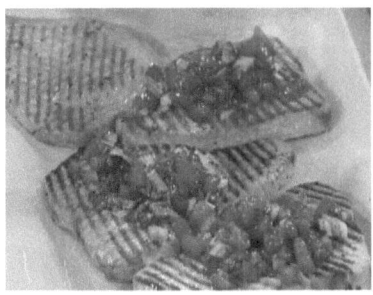

Fresh tuna steaks seasoned with coriander gives this dish a unique flavor. A rich ginger and garlic flavored tomato sauce complements the dish well. The touch of lemon juice and coriander infuses fresh flavors into the dish.

Ingredients

- 6 oz. of fresh tuna steaks
- 1 tsp coriander powder
- Salt and pepper for seasoning
- 2 tbsp. olive oil
- 1/2 cup chopped onions
- 1/2 cup chopped tomatoes
- 1 tsp minced garlic
- 1 tbsp. chopped coriander leaves
- 1 tsp lemon juice

Method

1. Marinate tuna with salt, pepper, and coriander powder. Drizzle olive oil on the fish and grill till done. This takes 1-2 minutes for a medium done steak.

2. Heat olive oil in a pan and cook all the remaining ingredients seasoned with salt and pepper except lemon juice and chopped coriander.

3. Place grilled tuna on a plate and pour the prepared sauce over the fish. Garnish with lemon juice and coriander leaves.

3 Benefits of Eating Tuna

Tuna is regarded as one of the world's healthiest food. Tunas are a rich source of omega-3 fatty acids that help maintain ideal weight and prevent the risk of cardiac diseases.

5. Rosemary-Garlic Lamb

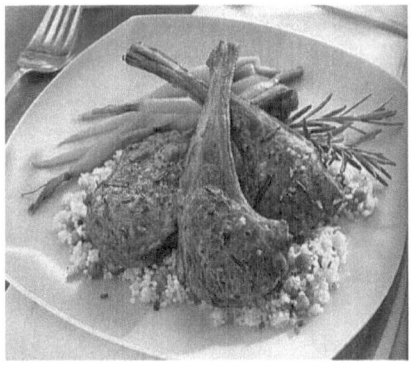

Lamb pieces are marinated in a mixture of spices and hung curd to add a unique flavor to the dish. The marinated meat is cover cooked with little a olive oil making the dish healthy.

Ingredients

- 1 1/2 cup chopped boneless lamb
- 1 tbsp rosemary
- 1 tbsp garlic paste
- 1 tsp pepper powder
- Salt as per taste
- 2 tbsp hung curd
- 1 tbsp lemon juice
- 1 tbsp olive oil

Method

1. Marinate lamb pieces with all the ingredients and set aside for 1 hour.

2. Heat olive oil in a skillet and add the marinated lamb pieces. Fry for few minutes. Cover and cook till done. The meat temperature will reach a temperature of 130F when the lamb is cooked to medium.

Cooking Tip

Lamb pieces can be marinated with the spices and stored in the refrigerator a day ahead for easy cooking.

Read This FIRST - 100% FREE BONUS

FOR A LIMITED TIME ONLY – Get Olivia's best-selling book *"The #1 Cookbook: Over 170+ of the Most Popular Recipes Across 7 Different Cuisines!"* absolutely FREE!

Readers have absolutely loved this book because of the wide variety of recipes. It is highly recommended you check these recipes out and see what you can add to your home menu!

Once again, as a big thank-you for downloading this book, I'd like to offer it to you *100% FREE for a LIMITED TIME ONLY!*

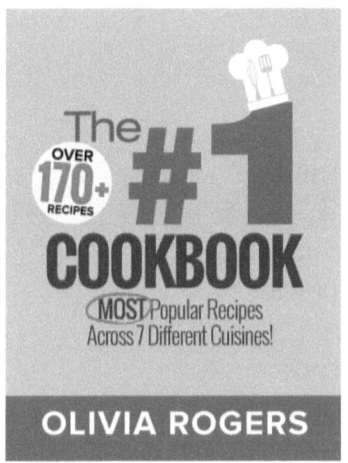

Get your free copy at:

TheMenuAtHome.com/Bonus

6. Cooked Lentil with Red Grapes and Mint

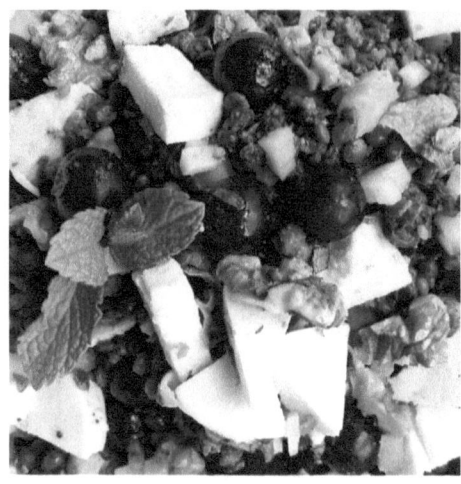

This wholesome recipe is a mix of cooked lentils tossed with fresh red grapes and toasted almonds. Chopped parsley and mint leaves adds a fresh taste to the dish.

Ingredients

- 1 cup cooked lentils
- 1 tbsp. olive oil
- 1 tbsp. sherry vinegar
- 1 tsp mustard powder
- Chopped leeks
- 1/2 cup red grapes
- 1 tbsp. toasted almonds
- Finely chopped parsley and mint leaves
- Salt as per taste

Method

1. Heat olive oil in a pan and sauté chopped leeks. Cook till they become soft. Remove from heat and add vinegar and mustard powder.

2. In a larger mixing bowl add the cooked leeks. Toss in the remaining ingredients and mix well.

Power Food Lentils

Lentils are a powerhouse of proteins and vitamins. These small seeds are high in nutritional value, low in sodium, and low in fat making them great for your health.

7. Mediterranean Greek Chicken Vegetable Salad

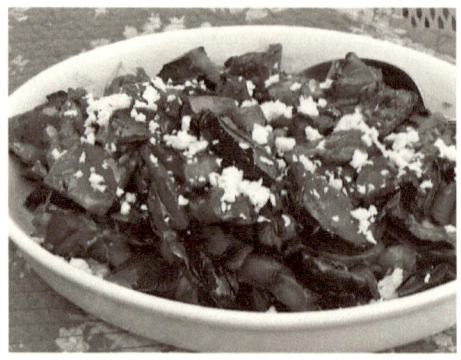

This Mediterranean Greek Salad is packed with fresh vegetables and boiled chicken pieces tossed in a flavorful low-fat salad dressing making it a wholesome meal.

Ingredients

For dressing

- 2 tbsp. of extra-virgin olive oil
- 1/3 cup of red wine vinegar
- Salt as per taste
- 1/4 tsp pepper powder
- Garlic powder
- 1 tbsp. chopped dill
- 1/2 cup feta cheese crumbled

Other ingredients

- 5 cups chopped iceberg lettuce
- 2 cups chopped boneless cooked chicken pieces marinated to taste (boiled)
- 1 cup chopped shallots
- 1/2 cup black olives

Method

1. Whisk the dressing ingredients in a bowl to form the salad dressing. In a bowl, combine lettuce, shallots, olives, and chicken and toss with dressing.

8. Grilled Salmon with Olive Oil and Rosemary

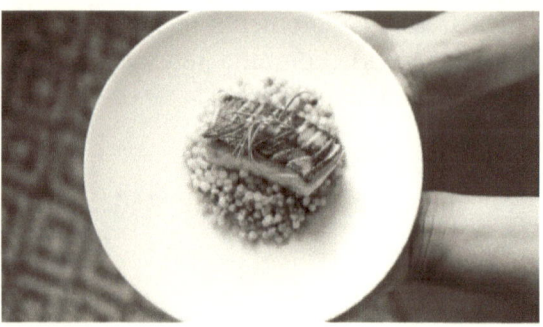

Salmon marinated with fresh rosemary is grilled on medium heat drizzled with a generous dose of olive oil to make this mouthwatering yet healthy recipe.

Ingredients

- 1-inch cubed salmon fillets
- 2 tbsp. olive oil
- 2 tsp fresh rosemary finely chopped
- 1 tsp lemon juice
- 1 tsp lemon zest
- 1/2 tsp salt
- 1/4 tsp pepper powder
- 1/2 cup cherry tomatoes

Method

1. Add all the ingredients in a large bowl, except olive oil, and toss well to marinate salmon and tomatoes. Arrange salmon and tomatoes on a skewer. Drizzle with olive oil and grill till cooked

Cooking Tip

Marinate the skewers and refrigerate for 8 to 9 hours to make delicious ready to cook skewers.

9. Grilled Tuna with Olive Dressing

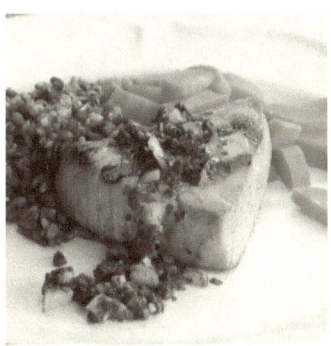

Generous amount of olive oil is whisked with garlic, oregano, and celery to create a great dressing for grilled tuna. This super easy recipe keeps you healthy and in shape.

Ingredients

- 4 tbsp. olive oil
- 1 tsp chopped celery
- 1 tsp minced garlic
- 1/2 tsp dried oregano
- 1 tbsp. lemon juice
- 1/2 tsp pepper powder
- 1 tsp salt
- 1 1/2 lbs. tuna steak

Method

1. Marinate tuna steak with all the ingredients and drizzle with olive oil. Heat grill and cook tuna till done. This takes 1-2 minutes for a medium done steak.

Cooking Tip

To make ready to cook tuna skewers, marinate tuna with all the ingredients and refrigerate for 8 hours.

10. Sardine and Chickpea Greek Salad

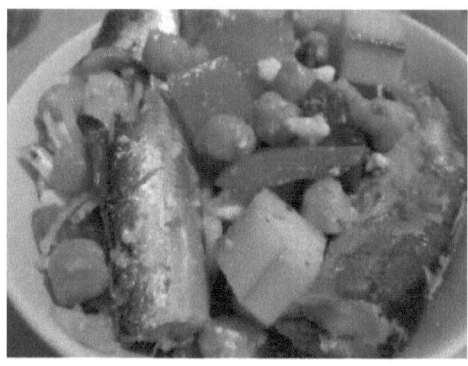

This low fat tangy salad is a yummy combination of lemon juice, cucumber, garlic, tomatoes, and olives. Chick peas, feta cheese and rich sardines all in a single salad bowl to keep you healthy and slim.

Ingredients

- 4 oz. can sardine
- 3 tbsp. lemon juice
- 1/2 cup chopped cucumber
- 1/2 cup chopped tomatoes
- 1/4 cup olives
- 1 tsp minced garlic
- 1/4 cup sliced red onion
- 3/4 cup boiled chick peas
- 1 tbsp. olive oil
- 1 tsp pepper powder
- 2 tbsp. crumbled feta cheese
- Salt as per taste

Method

1. In a bowl, sardines, lemon juice, cucumber, tomato, olives, garlic, red onion, chickpeas, oil, pepper powder, feta cheese, and salt. Toss well to coat.

3 Incredible Health Benefits of Sardines

Sardines are rich source of omega-3 fatty acids, vitamin D, and vitamin B12 essential for healthy heart, healthy skin, and healthy bones.

11. Spaghetti with Cottage Cheese

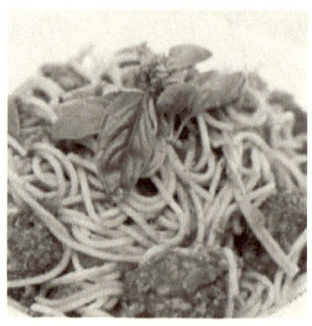

This Italian dish made with whole-wheat spaghetti and cottage cheese is complimented with a rich flavorful tomato sauce. The high fiber and protein rich dish complements your health as well.

Ingredients

- 8 oz. of whole wheat spaghetti
- 1 cup cubed cottage cheese
- 1 tbsp. olive oil
- 1 tbsp. minced ginger
- 1/2 cup chopped green bell pepper
- 1 cup chopped tomatoes
- Salt and pepper for seasoning
- 1 tsp oregano

Method

1. Cook pasta as per package instructions. Heat olive oil in a skillet and sauté ginger. Add bell pepper and fry while stirring.

2. Add tomatoes, seasoning ingredients, and oregano. Cook to make a thick sauce. Add cubed cottage cheese. Top the cooked spaghetti with prepared sauce.

12. Tangy Chickpeas Salad

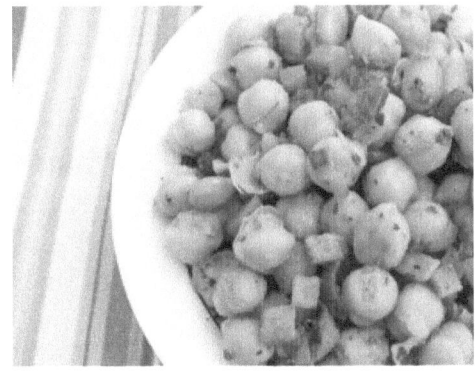

Boiled chickpeas tossed in a tangy and flavorful dressing to instantly create a healthy chickpea salad.

Ingredients

- 1 cup boiled chickpeas
- 1 tbsp. lemon juice
- 1 tbsp. chopped coriander leaves
- 1/2 cup chopped tomatoes
- 1/2 cup chopped cucumber
- 1/2 tsp salt

Method

1. In a large salad bowl, add chickpeas, lemon juice, coriander, tomato, cucumber, and salt. Toss well to coat.

13. Mediterranean Burger

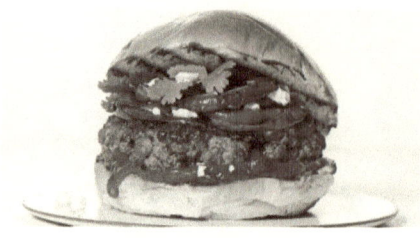

This healthy burger is made with lean meat and a mix of fresh seasoning topped with sour cream.

Ingredients

- 2 burger buns
- Sour cream
- Filling ingredients
- 1 large egg white
- 1 cup ground lean meat
- 1 tbsp. minced garlic
- 1 tbsp. minced ginger
- 1 tsp pepper powder
- Salt for seasoning
- 1/3 cup bread crumbs
- 1 tsp dry dill
- 1 tbsp. olive oil

Method

1. Mix all the filling ingredients in a bowl and shape into patties. Heat oil in a pan and cook patties. This usually takes on average 15 minutes.

2. Cut burger buns into halves. Place patties on buns with a spoonful of sour cream and cover with the other bun halves.

Store Patties

To store patties, place uncooked patties in air airtight container and store in the freezer.

14. Healthy Peanut Salsa

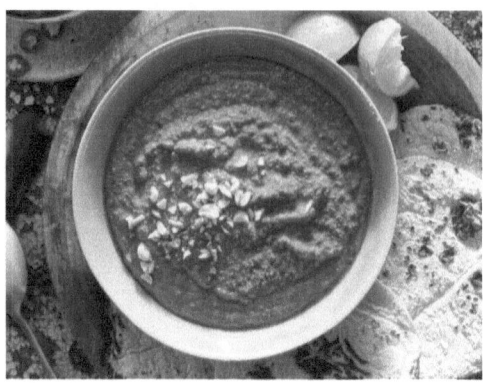

This spicy and tangy peanut salsa tossed with fresh herbs and seasonings goes well with multigrain bread or pitta bread.

Ingredients

- 1 cup boiled peanuts
- 1/4 cup chopped tomatoes
- 1/4 cup chopped English cucumber
- 1/4 cup chopped lettuce
- 1 tbsp. lemon juice
- 1 tbsp. chopped celery
- 1 tsp olive oil
- 2 slit green chilies

Method

1. In a bowl, add peanuts, tomato, cucumber, lettuce, juice, celery, oil, and chilies. Toss to coat.

15. Plum Tomatoes and Feta Cheese Salsa

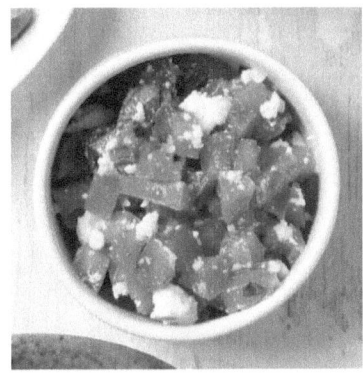

Plum tomatoes and feta cheese are tossed in a red wine dressing to make an amazing quick salsa.

Ingredients

- 1 cup chopped plum tomatoes
- 1/2 cup crumbled feta cheese
- 1 tsp dry oregano
- 1 tsp chopped basil leaves
- 1/2 tsp salt
- 1 tbsp. red wine
- 1 tbsp. toasted almonds

Method

1. In a bowl add, tomato, feta cheese, oregano, basil, salt, red wine, and toasted almonds. Serve with tortillas.

Tomatoes for Health

Tomatoes are a rich source of carotenoids that help fight against cancer. They are also an excellent source of vitamin C, which aids in eye health.

16. Gluten-Free Corn Salad

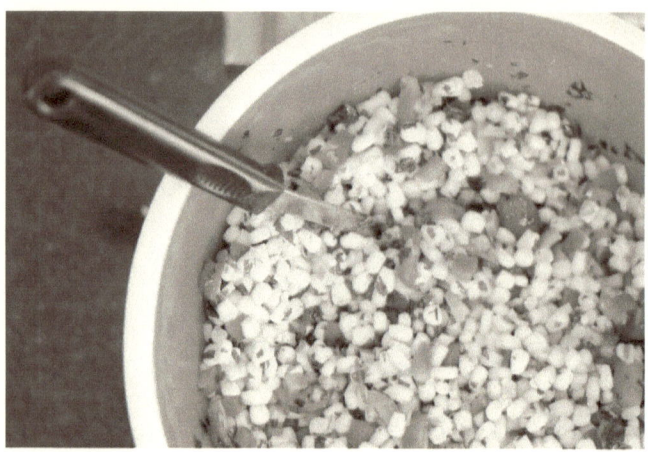

This delicious corn salad is prepared with freshly boiled sweet corn tossed with crumbled feta cheese, plum tomatoes, and black olives for a healthy brunch.

Ingredients

- 1 cup boiled sweet corn
- 1/2 cup crumbled feta cheese
- 1 cup chopped plum tomatoes
- 5 sliced black olives
- 1 pinch salt

Method

1. In a large bowl mix sweet corn, feta cheese, tomato, olive, and salt. Serve with pitta chips.

17. Roasted Bell Peppers and Zucchini Salad

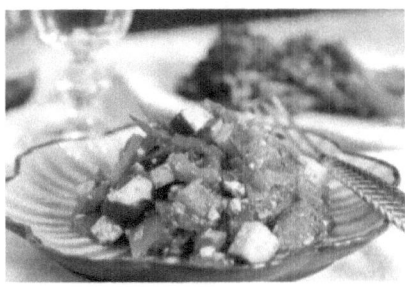

This nutritious salad is an assortment of sweet roasted bell peppers, juicy zucchini, plum tomatoes, and a mix of herbs drizzled with extra virgin olive oil.

Ingredients

- 1 1/2 cup sliced roasted bell peppers
- 1 cup chopped zucchini
- 1/2 cup chopped plum tomatoes
- 1 tbsp. finely sliced purple onions
- 1 tbsp. chopped basil
- 1 tsp capers
- A pinch of black pepper powder
- 1 tsp lemon juice
- 2 tsp extra virgin olive oil
- A pinch of salt

Method

1. In a large mixing bowl, add bell pepper, zucchini, tomato, onion, basil, capers, black pepper powder, lemon juice, oil, and salt. Toss to coat.

18. Plum Tomatoes and Feta Cheese Salsa

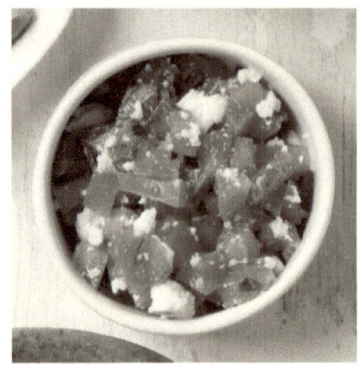

This super easy juicy salsa is a combination of plum tomatoes, feta cheese, and kalamata olives tossed with lemon juice and pepper powder.

Ingredients

- 2 cups diced plum tomatoes
- 1 cup of crumbled feta cheese
- 1/2 cup chopped kalamata olives
- 1/2 cup chopped parsley
- 1 tsp lemon juice
- 1 tsp pepper powder
- Salt to taste

Method

1. In a bowl, tomato, feta cheese, olives, parsley, lemon juice, pepper powder, and salt. Serve with whole-wheat crackers.

Useful Tips

This juicy salsa can be prepared ahead and stored in the refrigerator for up to 8 hours. Add salt and pepper just before serving.

19. Grilled Chicken Salad

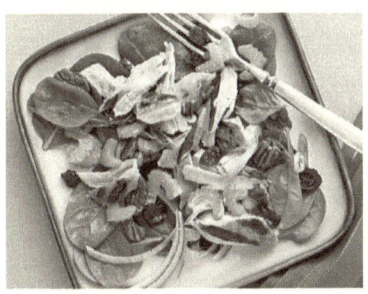

Grilled chicken tossed in roasted bell peppers and dried tomatoes with a mix of seasonings gives this salad a sweet and sour flavor for a healthy palate.

Ingredients

- 1 cup chopped grilled chicken
- 1/4 cup chopped roasted bell peppers
- 1/4 cup chopped dried tomatoes
- 1/4 cup chopped olives
- 1/4 cup feta cheese
- 2 tbsp. olive oil
- 1 tbsp. apple cider vinegar
- 1/4 cup chopped parsley
- Salt and pepper to taste

Method

1. In a large salad bowl, add chicken, roasted bell pepper, tomato, olives, feta cheese, oil, vinegar, parsley, and salt. Toss to coat.

Cooking Tip

Grilled chicken can be replaced with poached chicken to make an instant healthy salad.

20. Garden Fresh Mediterranean Salsa

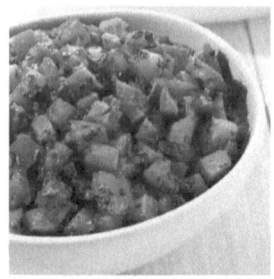

This fresh and healthy Mediterranean salsa is an assortment of garden fresh vegetables tossed with a fresh dash of lemon juice and chopped cilantro for refreshing flavors.

Ingredients

- 1 cup diced plum tomatoes
- 1/2 cup diced bell peppers
- 1/2 cup grated radish
- 1/2 cup sliced shallots
- 1/2 cup sliced black olives
- 1/4 cup sliced jalapeno
- 4 tbsp. chopped parsley
- Juice of 1 lemon
- Salt to taste

Method

1. In a bowl, add tomato, bell peppers, radish, shallots, olives, jalapeno, parsley, lemon juice, and salt. Serve with multigrain bread toast.

Useful Tips

Include fresh vegetables such as purple cabbage, cucumber, and add a handful of sprouts to transform this salsa to a nutritious meal.

21. Couscous with Cottage Cheese

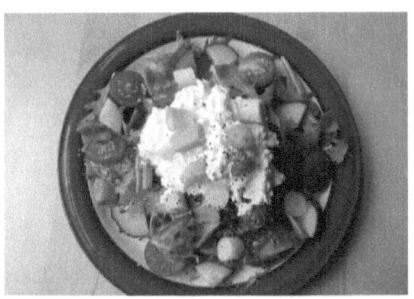

This delicious and low-fat couscous is prepared with cottage cheese, black olives, and chopped tomatoes for a juicy texture. Freshly squeezed lemon juice adds an extra zing to the dish.

Ingredients

- 1 cup of whole wheat couscous
- 1 1/2 cup of low sodium vegetable broth
- 1/2 cup grated cottage cheese
- 1/4 cup chopped cilantro
- 1/2 cup pitted and halved black olives
- 1/2 cup chopped tomatoes
- Salt and pepper to taste
- 1 tsp lemon juice
- 2 tbsp. extra virgin olive oil

Method

1. In a large pot, bring vegetable broth to boil. Stir in all the ingredients except lemon juice and cook over medium heat stirring in between. Add lemon juice, stir well and serve.

Cooking Tips

Finely sliced greens such as spring onions or spinach can be added to enhance flavor and increase nutritional value of this recipe.

22. Fruit and Cream Mexican Roll

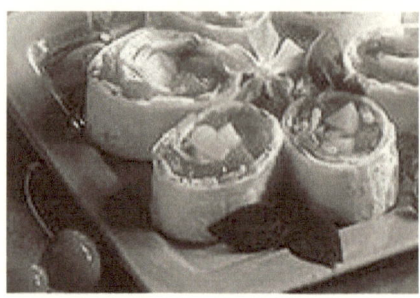

These yummy yet low fat creamy fruit rolls make a perfect start for a healthy breakfast.

Ingredients

- 1/2 cup low fat mayonnaise
- 1/2 cup low fat cheese cream
- 1/2 cup fine sliced pineapples
- 1/2 cup fine sliced apples
- 1 tsp sugar
- A pinch of salt
- 8 tortillas

Method

1. Mix all ingredients in a bowl. Spread the mixture on tortillas and roll them up. Refrigerate for a few hours and serve.

Useful Tip

Finely sliced fresh seasonal fruits such as strawberries and ripe bananas can also be added to the cream mixture as per taste.

23. Black Olives and Corn Mexican Cream Roll

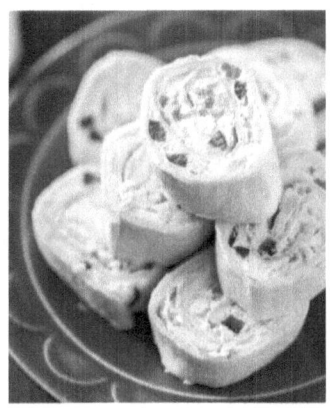

This delicious Mexican cream roll is filled with a mixture of low fat dressing blended with black olives and sweet corn for nutritious snack.

Ingredients

- 1 cup sour cream
- 1 cup cream cheese
- 1/4 cup sliced black olives
- 1/4 cup boiled sweet corn
- 1 tsp fresh pepper powder
- 1/2 cup grated cheddar cheese
- 4 flour tortillas

Method

1. Mix all ingredients in a bowl. Spread mixture over tortilla, and roll them up. Refrigerate for a few hours and serve.

24. Assorted Corn Macaroni Salad

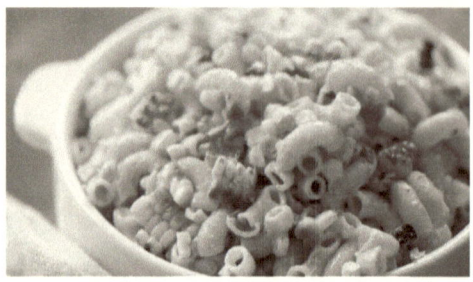

This Corn Macaroni Salad is an assortment of ingredients tossed with cooked macaroni and drizzled with a low-fat dressing.

Ingredients

- 2 cups cooked macaroni
- 1/2 cup boiled sweet corn kernels
- 1 cup cooked black beans
- 1 cup halved cherry tomatoes
- 1/2 cup chopped black olives
- 1/2 cup chopped cilantro

For dressing

- 1 cup spicy salsa
- 1 cup sour cream
- 1 tbsp. low fat mayonnaise
- 1 tsp white pepper powder
- Salt to taste

Method

1. Whisk together dressing ingredients in a bowl.

2. In a bowl combine, macaroni, corn, beans, tomato, olives, and cilantro. Add dressing to mixture, toss to coat, and serve.

Cooking Tip

Assorted macaroni salad can be prepared with fresh seasonal vegetables of your choice. This dish can be prepared ahead and refrigerated for a ready to serve meal.

25. Toasted Quinoa with Tomatoes and Parsley

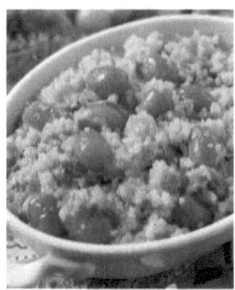

Roasted quinoa is cooked with tomatoes and a sprinkle of cumin powder for a superior flavor. This super food recipe is a great way to kick-start your day.

Ingredients

- 1 cup quinoa
- 1 tbsp. olive oil
- Cumin powder
- 1 cup chopped tomatoes
- 1/4 cup chopped parsley
- Salt to taste

Method

1. Toast quinoa to golden brown, and then cook with 1 cup water. Heat olive oil in a pan and sauté tomatoes. Add cumin powder, salt and fry well.

2. Pour cooked quinoa into the pan and sauté for a few more minutes. Garnish with chopped parsley

Super Food Quinoa

Quinoa is regarded as a one of the best sources of protein. Consumption of quinoa reduces weight and provides the body with essential nutrition such as vitamin E and phosphorous.

26. Beet and Fennel Salad with Low Fat Dressing

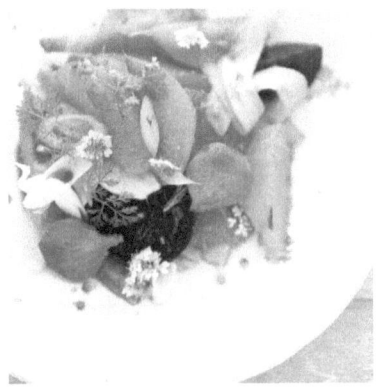

Boiled beets and fennel is tossed in a low-fat dressing to make this delicious and healthy salad.

Ingredients

- 1/2 cup sliced fennel heads
- 1 cup chopped beets (boiled)
- 1/2 cup bean sprouts

For dressing

- 3 tbsp. Greek yogurt
- 1 1/2 tbsp. apple cider vinegar
- 1 tsp olive oil
- 1 tsp brown sugar

Method

1. Whisk the salad dressing in a small bowl.

2. Place the vegetables and sprouts in a large bowl. Pour in the salad dressing and toss well to coat.

3 Incredible Benefits of Beets

Beets are highly nutritious and loaded with antioxidants, Vitamin A, and B complex vitamins are helpful for a healthy heart and aid in preventing cancer.

27. Mediterranean Fish Stew

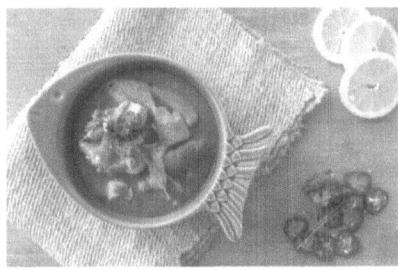

Thyme and orange rind add a little something extra to this dish to make it tasty and refreshing.

Ingredients

- 1 packet low sodium chicken broth
- 1 tbsp. olive oil
- 1 tbsp. fresh thyme
- 1 tsp coriander powder
- 1 tbsp. crushed garlic
- 1 tsp grated orange rind
- 4 saffron threads
- 1 pound of flounder fillet sliced into 2-inch strips
- Salt to taste

Method

1. In a large pot, add the chicken broth and bring to a boil.

2. Add the rest of the ingredients. Reduce heat and cook till fish turns soft.

Incredible Health Benefits of Flounder

Flounder is low in calories and high in proteins that help manage weight. It's also loaded with minerals and vitamins for a healthy heart and body.

28. Chopped Lamb with Lettuce

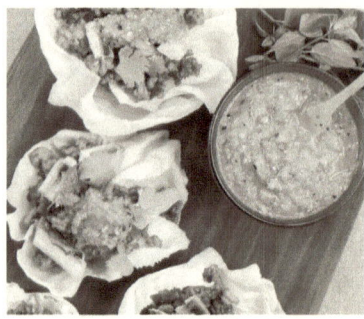

Minced lamp is covered and cooked on low heat with a mix of spices to make this delicious and low-calorie dish.

Ingredients

- 2 tbsp. olive oil
- 1 cup chopped lettuce
- 1 tbsp. ginger paste
- 1 cup minced lamb
- 1 tbsp. cinnamon powder
- 2 tbsp. chopped mint
- Chopped tomatoes
- 2 tbsp. chopped parsley
- 1 tsp pepper powder
- Salt to taste

Method

1. Heat oil in a skillet, and sauté all the ingredients except minced lamb. Add minced meat and season with salt. Cover and cook till meat becomes tender.

29. Spicy Grilled Shrimp

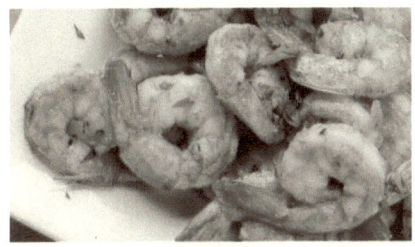

This delicious shrimp dish is marinated with an assortment of spices and grilled.

Ingredients

- 1 1/2 lbs. deveined medium size shrimps
- 2 tbsp. extra virgin olive oil
- 1 tsp cumin powder
- 1 tsp minced garlic
- 1 tsp paprika
- 2 tbsp. chopped cilantro
- 2 tbsp. chopped Italian parsley
- Juice of 1 lemon
- 2 tbsp. minced shallots
- Salt and pepper to taste

Method

1. Marinate shrimp with all ingredients and leave for at least 30 minutes.

2. Grill the shrimps till done. You can tell when the shrimp are done when their color loses its transparency, and curled into a "c" shape. If it has curled into an "o" shape it is over cooked.

3. Garnish with extra chopped cilantro and lemon juice.

30. Healthy Olive Mushroom Salad

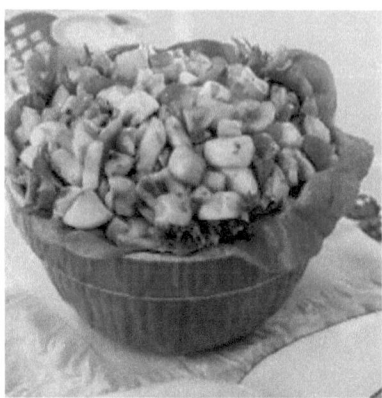

Olives are regarded as one the world's healthiest foods. They are loaded with healthy fats, antioxidants, and phytonutrients that protect the body from several diseases.

Ingredients

- 1 cup chopped Spanish olives
- 1/2 cup chopped red peppers
- 1/2 cup chopped lettuce
- 1/2 cup sliced cucumber
- 1 cup cooked and sliced mushrooms
- 1 cup vinaigrette dressing

Method

1. In a bowl add olives, red peppers, lettuce, cucumber, sliced mushrooms, and dressing. Toss well to coat.

31. Lemony Grilled Chicken

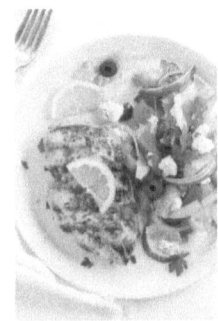

Chicken pieces drizzled with lemon juice and seasoned with paprika, cooked on the grill to make this juicy low-calorie chicken dish.

Ingredients

- 4 medium size chicken pieces
- 1 tbsp. lemon juice
- 1 tsp grated lemon rind
- 1 tbsp. paprika
- 1 tsp pepper powder
- 1 tbsp. olive oil
- Salt for taste

Method

1. In a bowl, add chicken, lemon juice, lemon rind, paprika, pepper powder, olive oil, and salt. Marinate the chicken for 30 minutes in this mixture.

2. Preheat your grill on medium-high heat. Place the chicken on the grill, and cook till done.

Cooking Tips

Chicken pieces can be replaced with tuna steaks to make lemony grilled tuna steaks.

32. Quinoa Salad with Lemon Garlic Dressing

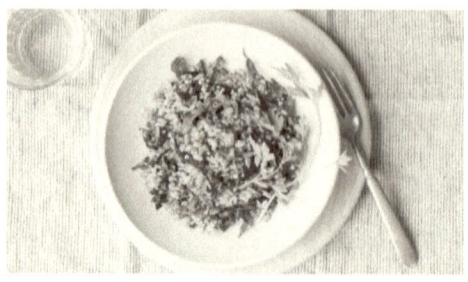

This is a healthy salad, which is quick and easy to prepare. It can be easily adapted to suit your own tastes by adding or removing your own choice of vegetables. This makes a delicious snack or meal, which can be eaten at any time of the day.

Ingredients

- Quinoa (cooked and chilled)
- Feta Cheese
- Black Beans (these should be rinsed and drained)
- Red peppers (finely chopped)
- Cherry tomatoes
- Cucumber
- Lettuce

Dressing

- Olive oil
- Lemon Juice (freshly squeezed)
- Pressed garlic clove
- Salt and pepper to taste

Method

1. In a bowl, combined your needed amount of quinoa, feta cheese, black beans, peppers, tomatoes, and cucumber.

2. To make dressing, whisk all the dressing ingredients together in a stainless-steel bowl.

3. Add dressing to salad bowl, toss to coat, and serve over a bed of lettuce leaves.

33. Quinoa Tabbouleh

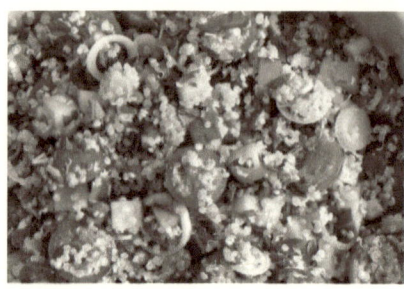

Quinoa is a grain which is high in fiber and protein. It is cooked in the same way as any rice dish, and has a mild flavor which makes it a perfect accompaniment to many dishes.

Ingredients

- 1 cup water
- 1/2 cup cooked quinoa
- 1/4 cup chopped tomatoes
- 1/4 cup fresh mint
- A little chopped cucumber
- 1/4 cup Raisins
- Dash of lemon juice
- 1 tbsp. of chopped onions
- 1/2 tbsp. of extra virgin olive oil
- Salt and pepper to taste

Method

1. The quinoa should be place into a saucepan with the water. This needs to be put on the stove and brought to the boil. It then needs to simmer for approximately 20 minutes; making sure that all the liquid is absorbed.

2. Next, fluff the quinoa with your fork and stir in the remaining ingredients.

3. Finally, you should cover the dish and leave it to stand for one hour. It can then be served at room temperature, or chilled if you prefer.

Top Tip

This dish is an excellent way of ensuring you have a healthy heart, enough fiber in your diet, and a serving has just 182 calories.

34. Beet, Blood Orange, Kumquat & Quinoa Salad

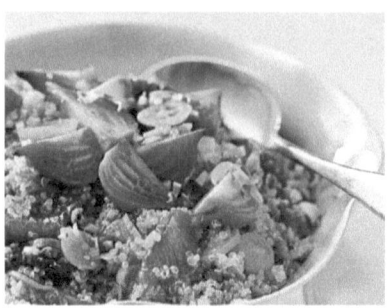

This is a citrus flavored salad, which blends a wide variety of flavors successfully creating an invigorating taste explosion. It is a colorful dish full of vitamins and proteins.

Ingredients

For the Dressing

- 1/4 cup green onions (chopped)
- 2 tsp grated blood orange rind
- 1 tsp grated lemon rind
- 2 tbsp. blood orange juice
- 1 tbsp. fresh lemon juice
- 2 tsp finely chopped cilantro
- 1/4 tsp salt
- 1/4 tsp ground coriander
- 1/4 tsp ground cumin
- 1/4 tsp paprika
- 3 tbsp. extra-virgin olive oil

For the Salad

- 1 cup uncooked quinoa
- 1 3/4 cups water
- 1/2 tsp salt

- 1 cup blood orange sections (chopped about 4 medium)
- 1 cup avocados (diced and peeled)
- 6 whole kumquats (seeded and sliced)
- 2 medium beets (cooked and cut into wedges)

Method

1. To make the dressing you will need to place all the ingredients in a bowl except for the oil. Once you have mixed or tossed the ingredients together you can slowly pour the oil into the bowl. Whilst doing this you need to be constantly stirring with a whisk.

2. Prepare the salad by placing the quinoa into a saucepan with the salt. Bring to the boil and simmer for approximately ten minutes. All the liquid should have been absorbed.

3. Next, remove this from the heat and fluff it gently with a fork.

4. Finally add all the ingredients and toss the mixture. Continue tossing the mixture whilst adding the dressing.

Health Facts

Quinoa is wheat free so it makes an excellent choice for cooking wholesome meals even if you suffer from gluten or allergy issues.

35. Chickpea Bajane

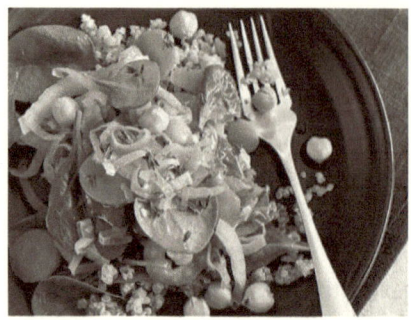

Bajane is actually a Provencal term used to describe the midday meal. Chickpeas are an essential part of the diet in this area and they are often stewed, making a delicious meal with pasta and vegetables. This is a variant of the traditional recipe.

Ingredients

- 2 tsp extra-virgin olive oil
- 1 garlic clove (minced)
- 1 cup organic vegetable broth
- 1 cup water
- 1 cup uncooked quinoa
- 1 1/2 tsp fresh thyme (chopped)
- 1/4 tsp salt
- 2 tsp extra-virgin olive oil
- 2 cups thinly sliced leek
- 4 garlic cloves (chopped)
- 2 1/2 cups sliced fennel bulb
- 1 3/4 cups carrot
- 1/2 tsp fennel seeds
- 1/2 cup white wine
- 1 cup organic vegetable broth
- 4 tsp chopped fresh thyme
- 1 can no-salt-added chickpeas; these will need to be rinsed and drained
- 1 tbsp. lemon juice

- 1/4 tsp salt
- 1/4 tsp freshly ground black pepper
- Baby spinach

Method

1. Firstly, you will need to prepare the quinoa; heat the oil in a large saucepan over a medium heat. Next add the garlic and sauté for a minute or two. Then add the broth, water thyme, quinoa and salt. Cover the dish, reduce the heat and allow the mixture to simmer for fifteen minutes.

2. To prepare the chickpea mixture you will need to heat some oil in the oven over a medium-high heat. Then, add the leek and 4 garlic cloves to the pan. This should then be sautéed for five minutes or until tender. You then need to add a little more oil, the fennel bulb, carrots and fennel seeds. This should be left to sauté for approximately ten minutes.

3. Finally, add the remaining oil, fennel bulb, carrot, and fennel seeds; sauté for a further ten minutes and the vegetables will go a golden-brown color.

4. Next add the wine and cook for a further three minutes or until liquid almost evaporates. Stir in the remaining broth, 2 teaspoons thyme, and chickpeas. Then cook for one minute or until thoroughly heated, then stir in the juice, 1/4 teaspoon salt, pepper, and spinach.

36. Cajun Crab & Quinoa Cakes

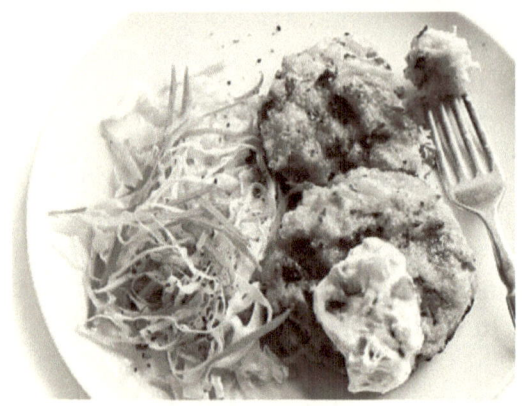

These Cajun spices add a little heat and flavor to this Mediterranean dish. Served with a little tartar sauce, you will get the right balance of spice and flavor.

Ingredients

- 4 cups water
- 1/2 cup uncooked quinoa
- 1 thyme sprig
- 1/2 tsp black pepper
- 1/2 tsp paprika
- 1/4 tsp ground red pepper
- 1/4 cup plain fat-free Greek yogurt
- 1/4 cup canola mayonnaise
- 1/4 cup chopped sweet pickles
- 1 tsp dijon mustard
- 8 oz. lump crabmeat (drained and shell pieces removed)
- 1/4 cup red bell pepper (chopped)
- 1/4 cup celery (chopped)
- 1/4 cup green onions (chopped)
- 1/2 cup kosher salt
- 1 large egg white
- 2 tbsp. olive oil

Method

1. Mix the first three ingredients in a saucepan and bring to a boil. Then simmer for thirty minutes or until mushy. Discard the thyme before draining. Allow it to cool slightly before moving on to the next step.

2. In a bowl, mix the black pepper, paprika, red pepper, yogurt, mayonnaise, pickles, and mustard. Place the crab in a bowl and mash slightly. Add the quinoa, spice mixture, and half of the yogurt mixture. Then stir gently whilst adding the egg white, red pepper, celery, green onions and salt.

3. Divide the mixture into 8 equal portions and gently pat into a 3-inch-wide patty. Then chill the patties for approximately 20 minutes. Preheat your broiler on high.

4. Line a pan with oil to avoid the patties sticking and arrange them on the pan. Then brush the tops with a little oil and sprinkle with some of the pepper mixture. Broil for approximately 5 minutes or until browned and then turn the cakes over and repeat the process on the other side.

37. Med Tuna Salad

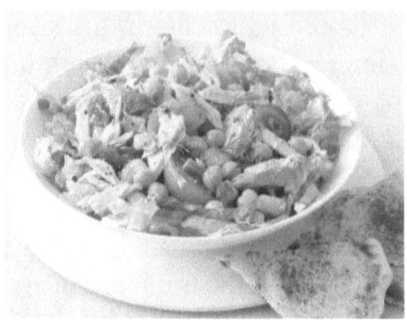

A quick and easy salad made with tasty tuna offers a variety of health benefits.

Ingredients

- 1 large can (12 ounces) water-packed solid albacore tuna (drained)
- 1 celery stalk, diced (1/2 cup)
- 1 strip (1 ½ inches) lemon zest, thinly sliced
- 3 tbsp. fresh lemon juice
- 3 tbsp. almonds, toasted and coarsely chopped
- 1 tbsp. and 2 tsp extra-virgin olive oil
- 2 tbsp. drained brine-packed capers, rinsed & coarsely chopped
- Coarse salt and freshly ground pepper
- ¼ cup dill sprigs
- 8 ounces mixed salad greens
- 4 slices multigrain bread (halved and toasted)

Method

1. Mix the tuna, diced celery, lemon zest, lemon juice, almonds, oil, capers, and ¼ teaspoon salt in a bowl.

2. Then season to your preferred taste with the pepper and stir gently. Add the dill and serve the tuna over greens. The bread

can be used to make toast, which makes a nice addition on the side.

Health Tip

Tuna is a one of the best sources of omega-3 fatty acids. Research suggests that these may protect against heart disease, high blood pressure, and many forms of cancer. Capers are an excellent source of antioxidants, which are essential to maintaining a healthy body.

38. Med Chicken Wrap

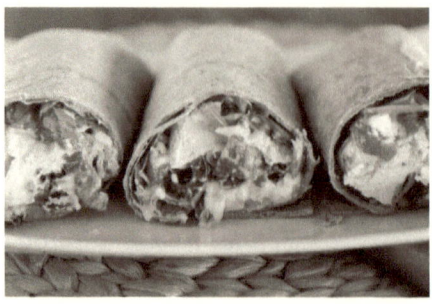

A simple, tasty, and filling snack, which will satisfy your taste buds at any time of the day.

Ingredients

- 1 chicken cutlet (3 oz.)
- Salt and ground pepper to taste
- 1 whole-wheat wrap
- 1 tbsp. olive tapenade
- 2 cans artichoke hearts (squeezed dry and thinly sliced)
- 1/2 small tomato (thinly sliced)
- 1/4 cup mixed baby greens

Method

1. Pre-heat your broiler ensuring the rack is four inches from the heat. Next, season the chicken with salt and pepper and broil until opaque throughout; this should take approximately four or five minutes. Leave the chicken to cool.

2. Now spread the bottom of the wrap with the olive tapenade. Add layers of chicken, artichoke hearts, tomato, and baby greens; season with salt and pepper to taste.

3. Finally fold tortilla to your desired shape and size, sealing the ingredients in.

Health Tip

Chicken is an excellent protein source and the tapenade adds several healthy fats. Artichoke hearts and tomato are both high in fiber, which are essential to any diet whilst the whole-wheat wrap will offer a better carb choice than a white wrap.

39. Chicken with Mustard, Greens, Olives, and Lemon

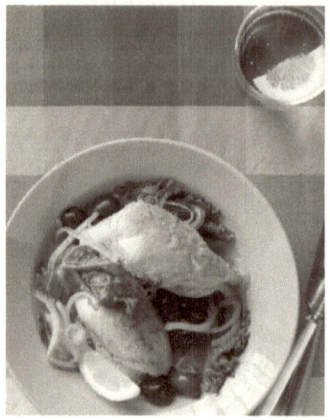

A tasty variant on the traditional chicken dish, which is guaranteed to have your taste buds singing!

Ingredients

- 2 tbsp. olive oil
- 6 chicken breast halves
- Salt and ground pepper
- 1 medium red onion (halved and thinly sliced)
- 4 garlic clove (crushed)
- 1 cup dry white wine
- 1 1/2 lbs. mustard greens (make sure you remove the stalks and coarsely chop the leaves)
- 1 tbsp. lemon juice.
- Lemon wedges are a nice addition for serving
- 1/2 cup pitted kalamata olives

Method

1. Start by heating a tablespoon of oil in a pot. While this is warming season your chicken with salt and pepper.

2. Add half of the chicken to the pot, and cook until browned on all sides. This should take between six and eight minutes. Place the cooked chicken on a plate and then repeat with the second half of your chicken pieces.

3. Now add onion and garlic to the pot, you may need to reduce the heat at this stage. Stir the onion and garlic until they soften then add the wine and chicken. Make sure you also add any juices, which have been generated along the way.

4. Bring the mixture to a boil. The pot now needs to be covered, and the heat reduced to a minimum. It should cook like this for approximately five minutes. Then add the greens on top of the chicken and season with salt and pepper, if necessary.

5. Cover and cook until chicken is opaque throughout and greens are wilted; this should be no more than another five minutes. Remove from the heat, and stir in lemon juice and olives.

Health Tip

Vitamin B12 is found in chicken and is an important nutrient for the body; it aids in the production of the soothing neurotransmitter GABA.

40. Stuffed Red Peppers

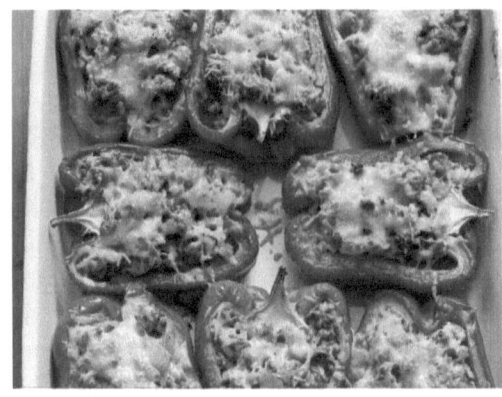

This is a simple yet tasty treat. It perfectly combines several flavors to give a unique taste of the Mediterranean.

Ingredients

- 4 red peppers
- 2 x 250g pouches tomato rice (cooked)
- 2 tbsp. pesto
- Handful of pitted black olives (chopped)
- 1/2 lb. goat's cheese

Method

1. Remove the tops from of the peppers, and scoop out all the seeds. Then place the peppers on a plate with the open top facing upwards. Then microwave on High for 5-6 minutes. Until they have wilted and softened.

2. While you are waiting for the peppers mix the rice with the pesto and olives and two-thirds of the cheese. Spoon the rice into the peppers, and put a little cheese on top.

3. Finally cook for between eight and ten minutes.

Health Tips

Red peppers contain as much as 300 percent of your daily vitamin C requirement. Vitamin C is also essential for the body to absorb iron correctly. Red bell peppers are high in vitamin A, which has been shown to help maintain healthy eyesight. Recent research has even suggested that sweet red peppers can activate thermogenesis whilst increasing your metabolic rate. This is essential for those who wish to lose weight.

41. Med Feta Salad with Pomegranate Dressing

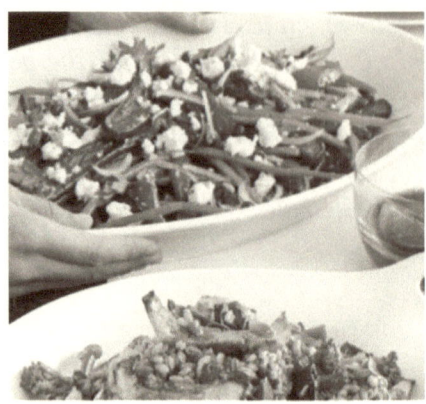

Pomegranates have long been known for their many health benefits. This recipe has a delicious way of combining them with a healthy salad. Enjoy the sunshine of the Med from wherever you are in the world.

Ingredients

- 2 red peppers
- 3 medium aubergines (these will need to be cut into chunks)
- 6 tbsp. extra-virgin olive oil
- 1 tsp cinnamon
- 200g green beans (blanched)
- 1 small red onion (sliced)
- 200g feta cheese (drained and crumbled)
- Seeds from 1 pomegranate
- Small amount of parsley

For the dressing

- 1 small garlic clove (crushed)
- 1 tbsp. lemon juice
- 2 tbsp. pomegranate molasses
- 5 tbsp. extra-virgin olive oil

Method

1. Pre-heat your oven to 200C/fan 180C/gas. Then turn the grill onto its highest setting and wait for it to heat up.

2. Cut the peppers into quarters before putting them on a baking sheet. They should be skin side up. Grill them until they are blackened. Place in a plastic bag, seal and then leave them for approximately five minutes. Wait until they have cooled, and then you will be able to scrape the skins off.

3. The aubergines need to be drizzled with olive oil, cinnamon, and seasoned with salt and pepper. Roast for roughly 25 minutes or until they are golden.

4. While they are cooking, mix all the dressing ingredients. Once the aubergines are ready place them with the green beans, onion, and peppers on a large serving plate, and sprinkle the feta and pomegranate seeds over the top.

5. Finally pour the dressing over top, and add a little parsley to garnish.

Health Tip

Pomegranates are rich in anti-inflammatory compounds, and have been shown to be very beneficial to those suffering from immune-related disorders like rheumatoid arthritis and osteroarthrits. Research has also shown that pomegranates assist in lowering blood pressure by preventing the activity of serum angiotensin-converting enzyme.

42. Orange, Anchovy, & Olive Salad

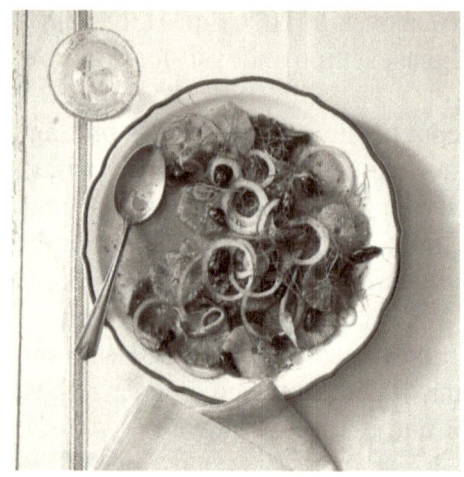

This surprising mix provides a delicate balance of flavors and a multitude of health benefits. Perfect for those who are looking to stay mentally as well as physically healthy.

Ingredients

- 4 small oranges
- 1 small red onion (sliced as thinly as possible)
- 16 black olives or Kalamata olives (pitted and halved)
- 6 anchovy fillets
- 1 tbsp. fresh lemon juice
- 3 tbsp. extra-virgin olive oil
- 1/8 tsp ground pepper to taste
- 2 teaspoons finely minced fennel fronds

Method

1. Carefully peel the oranges you should cut away all the white pith and the outer membrane. Then cut the oranges into thin slices; you should do this on a plate or bowl to catch as much of the juice as possible.

2. Place the orange slices on a serving dish, and save the juice. Place the onion over the oranges and arrange the olives over the top of the onion. Finally, the anchovy fillets should be put on top of everything else.

3. To finish pour the captured orange juice and the fresh lemon juice over the salad and drizzle with oil. Add pepper to taste. Ideally the salad should stay at room temperature for about half an hour; this will allow the flavor to soak through everything. Sprinkle the fennel fronds on the top to garnish.

Health Tips

Anchovies are known to contribute towards keeping your heart healthy, lower levels of bad cholesterol, and even help to keep toxin levels down. They have also been shown to help in improving skin health, reducing weight, and strengthening teeth. Meanwhile, olives have been shown to eliminate excess cholesterol in the blood, and to reduce the effects of degenerative diseases like Alzheimer's. They have even been known to assist those who are suffering with benign or malignant tumors, including varicose veins.

43. Spiced Turkey with Avocado/Grapefruit Relish

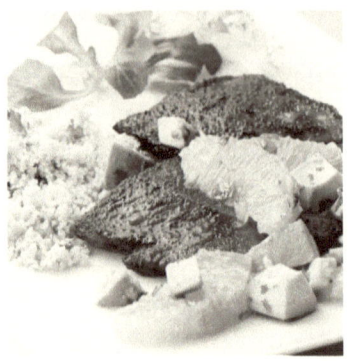

This dish combines the sharpness of the grapefruit, and the smooth taste of the avocado to perfectly balance the turkey, and make a mouth-watering meal.

Ingredients

- 1 large seedless grapefruit
- 1/2 small avocado
- 1 small shallot
- 1 tbsp. fresh cilantro (chopped)
- 1 tsp red-wine vinegar
- 1 tsp honey
- 1 tbsp. chili powder
- 12/ tsp five-spice powder
- Salt to taste
- 2 turkey cutlets
- 1 tbsp. canola oil

Method

1. Firstly, you should prepare the relish: Remove and discard the peel and white pith from the grapefruit. Then cut the segments from the grapefruit and allow them to drop into a small bowl. Squeeze any additional juice from the grapefruit

into the bowl. Next, add the avocado, shallot, cilantro, vinegar, and honey and toss them together.

2. You will then need to prepare the turkey: Combine the chili powder, five-spice powder, and a little salt on a plate. Roll the turkey in the spice mixture making sure it is fully coated.

3. Heat some oil in a medium skillet over medium heat. Once hot, add the turkey and cook for approximately two or three minutes. It should not be pink in the middle. Turn the turkey over and repeat on the other side. Then simply serve the turkey with the avocado-grapefruit relish.

Health Tip

Avocados increase the body's ability to absorb antioxidants from a variety of other foods. They are also high in antioxidants and potassium. Grapefruit is a natural food source, which helps to prevent constipation and encourages a healthy digestive tract.

44. Med Halibut Sandwiches

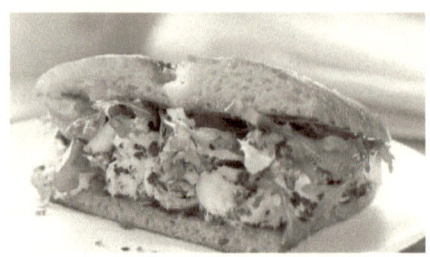

Fish has long been known to provide a myriad of health benefits and this recipe provides both a tasty way to enjoy it and a slight variant on the usual recipes.

Ingredients

- Vegetable oil cooking spray
- 2 halibut fillets (skinned)
- Salt and freshly ground black pepper
- Olive oil
- 1 loaf of ciabatta bread (This should be cut in half lengthways. You can remove the ends if you prefer)
- 1 garlic clove (halved)
- 1/3 cup mayonnaise
- 1/4 cup sun-dried tomatoes (chopped)
- 1/4 cup fresh basil leaves (chopped)
- 2 tbsp. fresh flat-leaf parsley leaves (chopped)
- 1 tbsp. capers (drained and mashed)
- Grated zest of 1 large lemon
- 2 cups arugula

Method

1. Preheat your oven to 450°C. Start by spraying a small baking dish with cooking spray, and then add the halibut and season with a pinch of salt and pepper according to your tastes.

2. Then rub each side of the halibut with a little oil. Cook this in the preheated oven until the flesh flakes easily with a fork. Leave it to cool.

3. Take the top half of the bread you previously sliced and brush the cut side with a little olive oil. Cool these for approximately 6 minutes until they are golden. You can then rub the toasted surfaces with garlic, according to your tastes.

4. Using a mixing bowl, you will need to combine the mayonnaise, sun-dried tomatoes, basil, parsley, capers, and lemon zest. Once this has been done add the flaked fish and mix. Spoon your mixture onto one half of bread and top with arugula.

5. Finally, place the top piece of bread on and cut into easily manageable sandwiches.

Health Tip

Halibut is rich in selenium; this is a mineral which is known to have antioxidant properties, and assist with regulating thyroid function. It also helps to ensure a healthy immune system.

45. Med Salmon

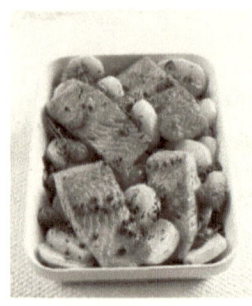

Salmon is a delicious fish that can be eaten in many different ways. This recipe combines the fish with a few simple vegetables to make a very healthy meal.

Ingredients

- 1/4 tsp salt
- 1/4 tsp black pepper
- 4 skinless salmon fillets
- Cooking spray
- 2 cups cherry tomatoes (these will need to be cut in half)
- 1/2 cup chopped zucchini
- 2 tbsp. capers (do not drain them)
- 1 tbsp. olive oil
- 1 can sliced ripe olives

Method

1. Your oven will need to be preheated to 425°C. The salmon should have salt and pepper sprinkled over both sides of it and then it can be placed into a baking dish coated with cooking spray.

2. Mix the tomatoes and all other ingredients in a bowl. Once it is fully mixed spoon it over the fish and cook for 22 minutes. Couscous can make an ideal addition to this dish.

46. Med Breakfast Couscous

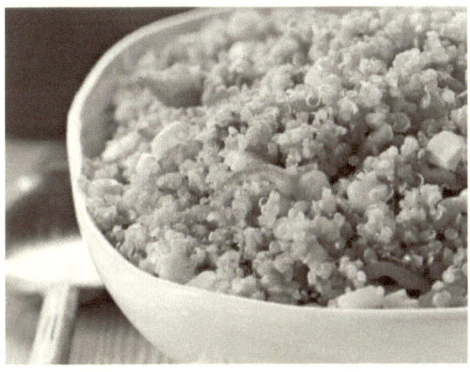

Couscous is an incredibly versatile dish, and can be combined with a wide range of ingredients to provide many different flavors. It is almost guaranteed

Ingredients

- 3 cups skimmed milk
- 1 cinnamon stick
- 1 cup uncooked whole-wheat couscous
- 1/2 cup chopped dried apricots
- 1/4 cup dried currants
- 6 tsp dark brown sugar
- Salt
- 4 tsp butter which will need to be melted

Method

1. Mix the milk and cinnamon stick in a pan over medium heat. Warm this until small bubbles form around the inner edge of the pan. Be careful not to boil or burn it.

2. Take the pan away from the heat and stir in couscous, apricots, currants, 4 teaspoons brown sugar, and salt. Cover mixture, and let stand for 15 minutes.

3. After 15 minutes the cinnamon stick can be discarded. The couscous should ideally be separated into 4 bowls, and each one should have a teaspoon of melted butter and 1/2 teaspoon of brown sugar drizzled on top of them.

47. Med Basmati Salad

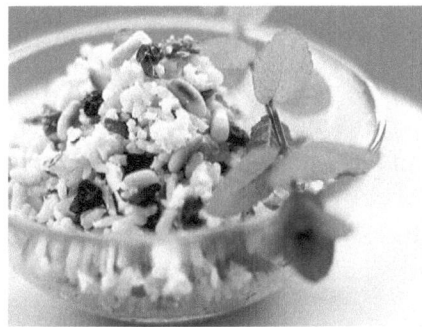

This is a quick and healthy salad with a delicate balance of flavors provided by pine nuts, currants and cheese. It is light and healthy.

Ingredients

- 2 sun-dried tomatoes
- 1/4 cup hot water
- 1 1/4 cups uncooked basmati rice
- 2 cups cold water
- 1/2 tsp salt
- 2.5 ounces feta cheese (crumbled)
- 2 tbsp. dried currants
- 2 tbsp. chopped fresh mint
- 1 tbsp. olive oil
- 1/4 tsp black pepper
- 2 tbsp. pine nuts (toasted)

Method

1. The tomatoes need to be left to stand for 10 minutes in a bowl of water; then chop them into small pieces. The rice goes into a separate bowl and needs to be covered with water to approximately two inches above the rice. Leave this to soak for 30 minutes, but be sure to stir occasionally. This will then need to be drained and rinsed.

2. Mix the rice and salt with two cups of water in a saucepan. Then bring this to a boil over medium heat, you will need to stir frequently to avoid it sticking or burning. Leave on the heat until the water level falls just below the rice.

3. Reduce the heat and allow to simmer for 10 minutes; then letting it stand and cool for 10 minutes. Spoon the rice into a bowl, and once it has cooled completely fluff it with a fork. Stir in the tomatoes, feta and the other ingredients except for the pine nuts; these should be sprinkled on top.

Health Tip

The fresh mint included in this recipe is an excellent source of vitamin A, which aids in good digestion. It is also helpful in making your breath smell nice.

48. Artichoke Provencal

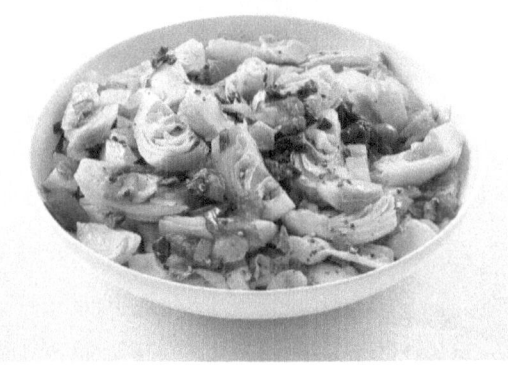

This recipe offers a taste of both France and the Med. It manages to merge a variety of flavors into a mouthwatering dish.

Ingredients

- 1/4 cup extra virgin olive oil
- 4 cloves garlic (crushed and peeled)
- Fresh thyme
- 1/2 cup black olives (pitted)
- Salt
- 12 little artichokes
- 1-pint grape tomatoes or about 1 1/2 cups any other tomatoes (chopped)
- Chopped fresh parsley

Method

1. Mix the oil and garlic in a large skillet over a low heat. Wait until the garlic sizzles then add herbs, olives, and a pinch of salt. Now prepare each of the artichokes by removing the hard leaves and cutting off the spiky ends; about an inch down from top. Trim the bottoms and cut the artichokes in half. Once they are ready place half of them into the pan.

2. Next, raise the heat to ensure the artichokes brown a little. Then add the remaining artichokes, and move them around to ensure they brown evenly.

3. Once they are brown add the tomatoes and a splash of water. Then cook until the artichokes are tender; this should take approximately 10 to 20 minutes. More water can be added if needed. Add seasoning and garnish to your own tastes and serve hot or at room temperature.

Health Tip

Artichokes are well known for their ability to detoxify the body. They have also been shown to improve the health of the liver and aid in resolving digestive issues like indigestion, constipation, Irritable Bowel Syndrome, and diarrhea.

49. Vegetable and Garlic Calzone

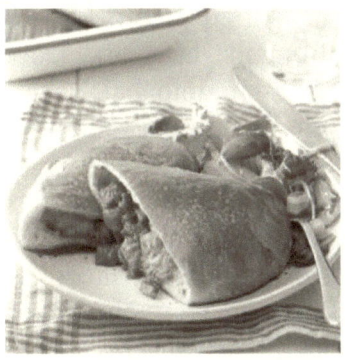

This is a delicious mixture of pastry and an assortment of healthy vegetables. This recipe is ideal for when you are looking for something a little different.

Ingredients

- 3 asparagus stalks (cut into 1-inch pieces)
- 1/2 cup chopped spinach
- 1/2 cup chopped broccoli
- 1/2 cup sliced mushrooms
- 2 tbsp. garlic
- 2 tsp olive oil
- 1/2-pound frozen whole-wheat bread dough loaf (thawed)
- 1 medium tomato (sliced)
- 1/2 cup mozzarella cheese (shredded)
- 1/2 cup pizza sauce

Method

1. Preheat the oven to 400 F, and then lightly coat a baking sheet with cooking spray. In a mixing bowl mix the asparagus, spinach, broccoli, mushrooms, and garlic. Then place 1 teaspoon of the olive oil over the vegetables, and toss to mix well.

2. Heat a large frying pan over medium-high heat. Next add the vegetables, and sauté them for approximately 5 minutes. They should be stirred frequently. When they are ready remove them from the heat, and leave to cool. The bread dough should be split into half, and each half should be pressed into a circle. Using a rolling pin, roll the dough into an oval.

3. On one half of the oval, add 1/2 cup of the sautéed vegetables, 1/2 of the tomato slices, and 1/4 cup of cheese. You will then need to wet your finger, and rub it over the edge of the dough that you have just filled. Place the other half of the dough on top of the other side (fold the dough basically in a half crescent) and roll the edges together.

4. Place the finished product onto a baking sheet ready for the oven. Make the second Calzone and brush them all with the remaining olive oil. Place the calzones in the oven for approximately 20 minutes. Bake until golden brown.

5. To serve you should heat the pizza sauce in the microwave. Then place each calzone onto a plate. Serve with 1/3 cup pizza sauce on the side or pour the sauce over the calzones.

Health Tip

Garlic is low in calories and very rich in Vitamin C, Vitamin B6, and Manganese. It also contains trace amounts of various other nutrients.

50. Tuscan White Bean Stew

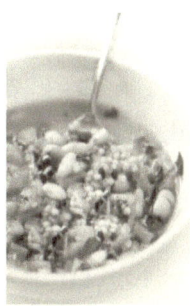

This is a heart-warming meal, perfect for those colder days when it is tempting to succumb to the call of comfort food.

Ingredients

- 1 tbsp. extra-virgin olive oil
- 2 cloves garlic (quartered)
- 1 slice whole-grain bread (cut into approximately ½ inch cubes)
- 2 cups dried cannellini (these need to be rinsed and then soaked overnight)
- 6 cups water
- Salt
- 1 bay leaf
- 2 tbsp. olive oil
- 1 yellow onion (chopped)
- 3 carrots (peeled and chopped)
- 6 cloves garlic (chopped)
- Freshly ground black pepper
- 1 tbsp. chopped fresh rosemary
- 1 1/2 cups vegetable stock

Method

1. First make the croutons by heating the olive oil in a large frying pan. Add the garlic and sauté for 1 minute. Then let it

stand for roughly 10 minutes. This will allow the flavor of the garlic to be absorbed by the oil. Now you can remove the garlic pieces, and return the pan to the heat.

2. Next the bread cubes will need to be sautéed, they should be stirred regularly until they are a golden brown. To make the soup choose a suitable pot and mix the white beans, water, some salt, and the bay leaf. Slowly bring this mixture to a boil, and then make sure the heat is as low as possible, this must be left to simmer for between 60 and 75 minutes.

3. You can then drain the beans; it is a good idea to reserve 1/2 a cup of the cooking liquid and make sure you remove the bay leaf. You will then need to form a paste from the reserved cooking liquid, and half the cooked beans. They should be mixed and mashed before adding them to the other beans.

4. Next add the olive oil and return to the heat. Stir in the onion and carrots and sauté until the carrots are tender-crisp before stirring in the garlic and heated for a further minute to soften the garlic.

5. Stir in a little more salt, pepper, chopped rosemary, bean mixture, and stock before bringing the entire mixture to a boil, simmer this for approximately 5 minutes to ensure it is heated thoroughly. Sprinkle the croutons on top when serving.

Health Tip

Cannellini beans are known to be full of antioxidants. It also takes longer for the body to digest these beans than most other foods, this will keep you feeling full for longer and provide a good flow of energy throughout the day.

51. Roasted Cod with Warm Tomato-Olive-Caper Tapenade

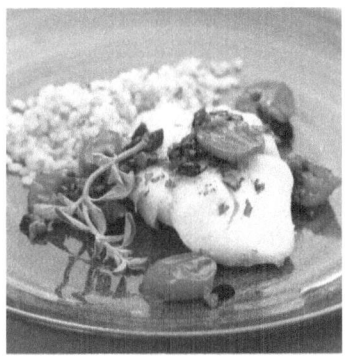

Fish is known to have many health benefits, and this recipe will provide you with a quick and simple way to enjoy these benefits.

Ingredients

- 1 lb. cod fillet
- 3 tsp extra-virgin olive oil
- Freshly ground pepper
- 1 tsp minced shallot
- 1 cup halved cherry tomatoes
- 1/4 cup chopped cured olives
- 1 tbsp. capers (rinsed and chopped)
- 1 1/2 tsp fresh oregano (chopped)
- 1 tsp balsamic vinegar

Method

1. Before starting you should prepare the oven by preheating it to 450°F, and coating a baking sheet with cooking spray. Take your cod and rub the oil into both sides before sprinkling with pepper. Place this on your baking sheet and roast until the fish flakes easily with a fork. This should take approximately 15 to 20 minutes.

2. While this is cooking you will need to heat a little oil in a small skillet, add the shallots and cook, keep stirring until they begin to soften. Next add the tomatoes and repeat; stirring until softened. Add your olives and capers and cook for a further thirty seconds.

3. Finally, stir in the oregano and vinegar and then spoon the mixture over the cod to serve.

Health Tip

Consuming White fish regularly has been shown to improve blood pressure. Research has also linked it with assisting to lower cholesterol, and has been shown to help people reduce weight.

52. Med Grilled Vegetable Tagine

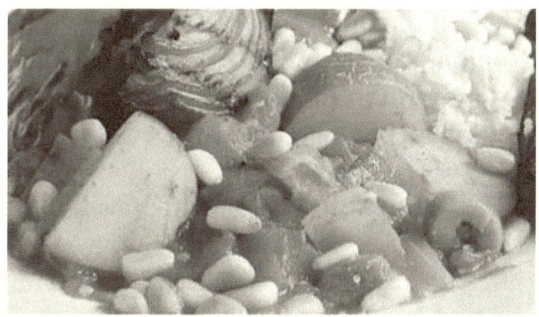

This delicious dish provides all the flavors of the med and combines them in a healthy way, which can be enjoyed at any time of the year.

Ingredients

- 1 small red onion
- 2 red bell peppers
- 1 green bell pepper
- 2 tsp balsamic vinegar
- Salt
- 1 tsp olive oil
- 1 3/4 cups chopped onion
- 2 garlic cloves
- 1 tsp ground cumin
- 1/2 tsp fennel seeds (crushed)
- 1/4 tsp ground cinnamon
- 1 1/4 cups water
- 1/4 cup sliced pitted green olives
- 1/4 cup raisins
- Freshly ground black pepper
- 1 can diced tomatoes (undrained)
- 6 small red potatoes
- Cooking spray
- 1/2 cup uncooked couscous
- 1/4 cup pine nuts (toasted)

Method

1. Cut the red onion into wedges but avoid cutting the end. Mix the red onion, bell peppers, vinegar, a pinch of salt, and a little oil in a zip-top plastic bag. Seal the bag and shale to mix, ensuring all the ingredients are coated in the oil.

2. Next, heat a little oil in a large skillet and add the onion and garlic; chopped. Allow the mixture to sauté for approximately 3 minutes. Then add the cumin, fennel, and cinnamon and sauté for a further minute.

3. Next you will need to add a little salt and 1/4 cup of water, olives, raisins, black pepper, tomatoes, and potatoes then bring the mixture to a boil. This will need to simmer for approximately 20 minutes to allow the potatoes to become tender. The marinated bell peppers and red onion now need to be grilled for approximately 10 minutes. They should be coated with the cooking spray and turned regularly.

4. Next you will need to cook the couscous by bringing a cup of water to a boil and gradually stirring in the couscous. It should then be allowed to stand for 5 minutes before being fluffed with a fork.

5. To serve pour the tomato mixture over the couscous, and top with the grilled bell peppers and red onions. Pine nuts can be sprinkled on top to taste.

Health Tip

There are plenty of heart-healthy fats and an impressive 14 grams of fiber in this stew. This delicious low-calorie meal will provide you with roughly half your daily-required amount of fiber.

53. Barley and Roasted Tomato Risotto

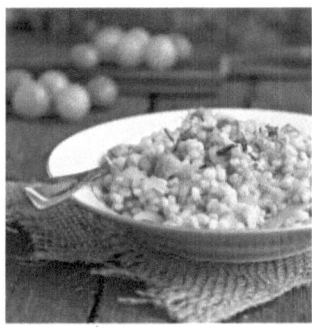

This is an excellent way of eating healthily while enjoying some varied flavors. This recipe can easily be customized to your own tastes.

Ingredients

- 10 large plum tomatoes (they need to be peeled and cut into 4 wedges)
- 2 tbsp. extra-virgin olive oil
- Salt
- Freshly ground black pepper
- 4 cups vegetable stock
- 3 cups water
- 2 shallots (chopped)
- 1/4 cup dry white wine
- 2 cups pearl barley
- 3 chopped fresh basil (plus whole leaves for garnish)
- 3 tbsp. fresh flat-leaf parsley (chopped)
- 1 1/2 tsp fresh thyme (chopped)
- 1/2 cup grated Parmesan cheese (plus a little extra for making curls to garnish)

Method

1. Place the tomatoes on a baking sheet; drizzle with the olive oil and sprinkle with a pinch of salt and 1/4 teaspoon of

pepper. Gently mix by tossing. This needs to be roasted until the tomatoes are softened and just beginning to brown. You will need 16 tomato wedges for the garnish.

2. Using a medium size saucepan mix the vegetable stock and water and bring it to a boil. This mixture should be left to simmer.

3. In a different saucepan heat the remaining olive oil and add the chopped shallots. Sauté until soft and translucent and then stir in the white wine. Continue to sauté until most of the liquids have evaporated.

4. Next, stir in the barley and 1/2 a cup of the stock mixture; cook until the liquid is completely absorbed. Slowly stir in the remaining stock mixture a little at a time. You need to make sure the majority of the liquid has been absorbed before adding more. Once all the moisture has been absorbed the barley should be tender. This process may take approximately 50 minutes. You will now need to take the pan off the heat, and fold in the tomatoes, chopped basil, parsley, thyme, and grated cheese.

5. Finally, stir in a little salt and pepper to taste. To serve the risotto should be placed into warm shallow bowls. This can be garnished with the reserved roasted tomato wedges, and the whole basil leaves. You can also add some curls of Parmesan cheese, if desired.

Health Tip

Barley is an excellent food for a variety of valuable nutrients; such as molybdenum, manganese, dietary fiber, and selenium. It is also rich in copper, vitamin B1, chromium, phosphorus, magnesium, and niacin.

54. Braised Kale with Cherry Tomatoes

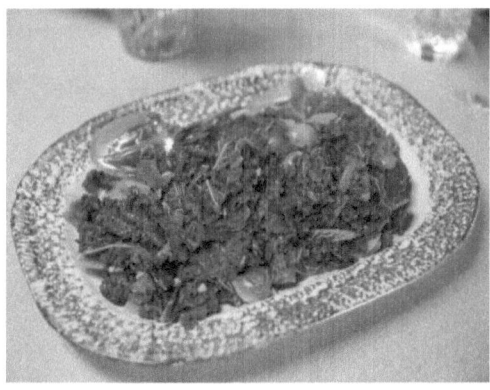

This is a simple meal, which can be made in just a few minutes and provides a nourishing, healthy and fulfilling meal at any time of the day.

Ingredients

- 2 tsp extra-virgin olive oil
- 4 garlic cloves (thinly sliced)
- 1 lb. kale (tough stems removed and leaves coarsely chopped)
- 1/2 cup vegetable stock
- 1 cup cherry tomatoes (these will need to be halved)
- 1 tbsp. fresh lemon juice
- Salt
- Freshly ground black pepper

Method

1. Place the olive oil in a pan, and add garlic; sauté until lightly golden.

2. Next you will need to stir in the kale and vegetable stock; this should all be covered and left for approximately 5 minutes to ensure the kale has wilted. You can then add the tomatoes

and cook, uncovered; it should take no longer than 7 minutes to ensure the kale is tender.

3. Take the pan off the stove, and add the lemon juice, salt, and pepper. This should be served immediately.

55. Roasted Eggplant and Feta Dip

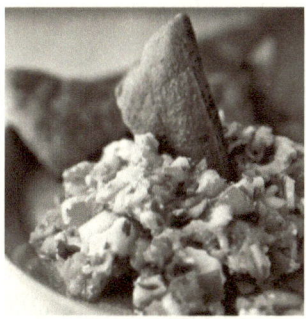

This recipe is a delightful concoction of onions, peppers, and cheese with the added kick of jalapeno. A taste explosion!

Ingredients

- 1 medium eggplant
- 2 tbsp lemon juice
- 1/4 cup extra-virgin olive oil
- 1/2 cup crumbled feta cheese, preferably Greek
- 1/2 cup red onion (finely chopped)
- 1 small red bell pepper (finely chopped)
- 1 small chili pepper, such as jalapeño, seeded and minced (this can be left out if not to your tastes.)
- 2 tbsp. fresh basil (chopped)
- 1 tbsp. flat-leaf parsley (finely chopped)
- Cayenne pepper
- Pinch of sugar if required

Method

1. The rack in your oven should be approximately 6 inches from the heat. Put the eggplant in a pan, and poke some holes in it to ensure that the steam can vent. Broil the eggplant; you will need to turn this every five minutes until the skin is charred.

2. To test you should insert a knife into the dense flesh near the stem. It should go in easily. Then place the eggplant on a cutting or cooling board until cooled.

3. Next, put lemon juice in a bowl and add the eggplant. This will need to be cut in half lengthways and the insides scrapped into the bowl.

4. Mix this with the lemon juice to ensure it is fully covered; this will prevent discoloring. You will then need to add a little oil, and stir until the oil is completely absorbed. Add the feta, onion, bell pepper, chili pepper, basil, parsley, cayenne, and salt. Sugar can be added if required.

56. Honey and Olive Oil Zucchini Muffins

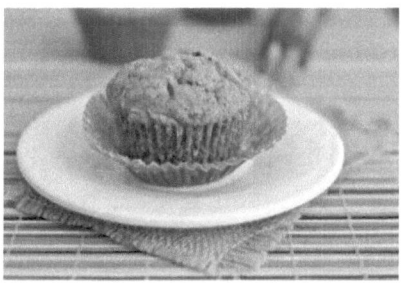

These muffins are a real treat; they are moist and deliciously sweet inside. They can be eaten at breakfast, lunch, and even as a bedtime treat!

Ingredients

- 3 cups zucchini (grated)
- 2 beaten eggs
- 2 tsp vanilla
- 1 cup olive oil
- 2/3 cup maple syrup
- 1/3 cup raw honey (softened)
- 1 1/2 cups whole wheat flour
- 1 1/2 cups all-purpose flour
- 2 tsp baking soda
- 2 tsp baking powder
- Salt
- 1 1/2 tsp cinnamon

Method

1. Firstly, combine the zucchini, eggs, vanilla, olive oil, maple syrup, and honey; these can be stirred gently together until mixed well.

2. In a separate mixing bowl, combine the whole wheat flour and all-purpose flour, baking soda, baking powder, salt, and

cinnamon. Mix thoroughly and then make a hole in the middle.

3. Pour the zucchini mixture into this hole and stir briefly. The ingredients should be barely combined. This is essential as over mixing will make the muffins hard.

4. Next pour the batter into a greased muffin tin. Alternatively, you can use paper cups.

5. The mixture will make approximately 8 jumbo muffins or 15 regular sized ones. These should be baked until they are golden brown. A further test can be performed by pressing gently on the top; they should spring back.

Health Tip

With only 17 calories per 100 grams the zucchini is a very healthy vegetable. It has no saturated fats or cholesterol and is even a good source of fiber. This can help reduce constipation and research suggests may offer some protection against colon cancers.

57. Arugula Salad with Cucumber, Feta, and Mint

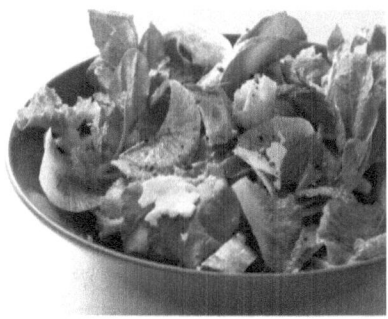

Bread with a salad of greens and tomatoes is not a new dish; it has been very popular in the Mediterranean for years. This recipe adds an additional twist by including some cucumbers, radishes, and olives.

Ingredients

- 4 to 6 fresh mint leaves (coarsely chopped)
- 6 tbsp. extra-virgin olive oil
- 1 1/2 tbsp. red wine vinegar
- Salt
- 1 1/2 ounces plain cracker or crisp bread
- 3 cups arugula
- 1 small cucumber (peeled and thinly sliced)
- 4 small radishes (trimmed and thinly sliced)
- 1/4 cup drained (crumbled feta cheese)
- Fresh black pepper
- 12 small black olives

Method

1. Place the mint, olive oil, and vinegar in a bowl and mix until you obtain a smooth dressing. Add a little salt to your required taste.

2. The cracker bread needs to be broken into small, bite-sized pieces and then put into the bottom of a salad bowl. Pour about one third of the dressing mix onto the crackers and add the argugula. Mix thoroughly.

3. Next, you will need to add the cucumber and radishes; then drizzle the rest of the dressing on top. Gently mix to ensure everything is covered with the dressing.

4. Finally, sprinkle the feta and any pepper on top and serve garnished with the olives. More oil or vinegar can be added if required.

Health Tip

Fresh mint contains powerful antioxidants, which assists in healthy digestion. It also helps to keep your breath fresh.

58. Arugula-Pear Salad with Parmesan and Walnuts

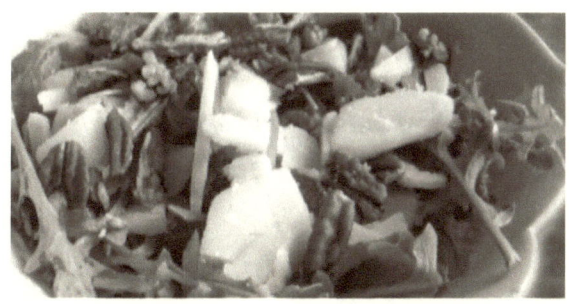

Adding a few simple ingredients can make this traditional salad. This is an excellent example of how simple it is to put together a tasty and nutritious meal.

Ingredients

- 8 cups trimmed arugula (washed and drained)
- 2 pears (these can be cut into 1-inch chunks)
- 1/2 cup walnuts (chopped)
- 4 oz. parmesan or Greek graviera cheese
- 4 tbsp. olive oil
- 2 tbsp. balsamic vinegar
- 1 tbsp. honey
- 2 tbsp. orange juice
- Salt and pepper
- 1/2 tsp cayenne pepper

Method

1. The arugula should be put into a mixing bowl with the chopped pears and half the Walnuts. This can be mixed and then set aside until the rest of the salad is ready.

2. In a different bowl, whisk the remaining ingredients until a smooth dressing is created. Pour the mixture over the

prepared salad and toss to coat. Using a vegetable peeler, shave the cheese into thin strips, and lay on top of the salad along with the rest of the walnuts.

Health Tip

Walnuts, eaten in moderation can add essential fats to your diet and actually help you to maintain your ideal weight.

59. Avocado Gazpacho

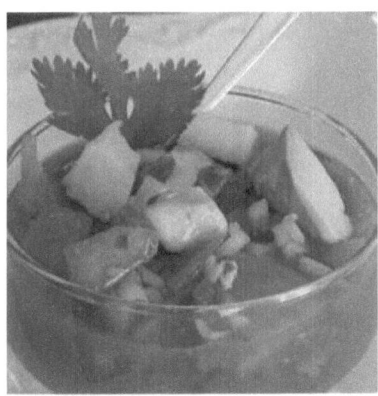

This is a very refreshing dish, and can be particularly delightful on a hot summer's day. To make the most of the flavors you should prepare this early, and allow it to chill for several hours.

It can easily be turned into a full meal by adding hard-boiled eggs, whole-grain croutons, diced bell peppers, and fresh chopped parsley or basil.

Ingredients

- 2 cups chicken or beef broth
- 1/2 cup fresh lemon juice
- 2 tbsp. extra-virgin olive oil
- 10 tomatoes (finely chopped)
- 1 1/2 large green bell peppers (finely chopped)
- 1 small red onion (chopped)
- 1 tbsp. paprika
- 1 clove garlic
- Salt and freshly ground pepper to taste
- ½ cucumber (this will need to be peeled, cut in half lengthwise and chopped)
- 1 large ripe avocado (seeded, peeled, and cut into 1-inch cubes)

Method

1. Mix the broth, lemon juice, olive oil, tomatoes, peppers, onion, paprika, garlic, salt, and pepper in a blender or food processor. You will need to pulse this until fully mixed, but with a few chunks remaining.

2. The mixture can be placed into one bowl or several individual bowls, and then needs to be chilled for several hours. If possible, leave it chilling overnight. When serving garnish with avocado and cucumber.

Health Tip

Avocados are rich in vitamins C, E, K, and B-6, which are all essential for a healthy body. It is also an excellent source of riboflavin, niacin, folate, pantothenic acid, magnesium, and potassium. They have been shown to be one of the healthiest foods you can eat.

60. Avocado-Watermelon Salsa

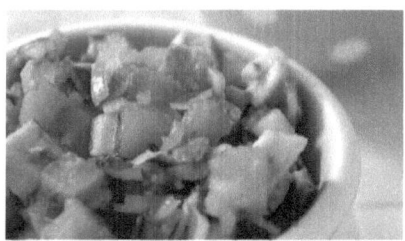

This salsa perfectly mixes the cool tastes with a little zing, and is a tasty dish for any occasion. It is best served with either corn or pita chips.

Ingredients

- 2 cups watermelon cubes
- 2 ripe avocados (peeled, seeded, and diced)
- 1 tbsp. fresh cilantro (minced)
- 1 tbsp. chopped jalapeño pepper (this can be replaced with red bell peppers if preferred)
- 1/2 cup green bell peppers (chopped)
- 2 tbsp. lime juice
- 1 tbsp. green onions (chopped)
- Garlic
- Salt to taste

Method

1. Place all ingredients in a mixing bowl, and mix thoroughly. It can be served immediately, but is better if left to chill for approximately 1 hour.

Health Tip

Watermelon is low in calories and has a surprisingly high level of various vitamins and minerals. It is also rich in antioxidants, and is a great addition to any diet.

61. Black Bean, Edamame, and Wheat Berry Salad

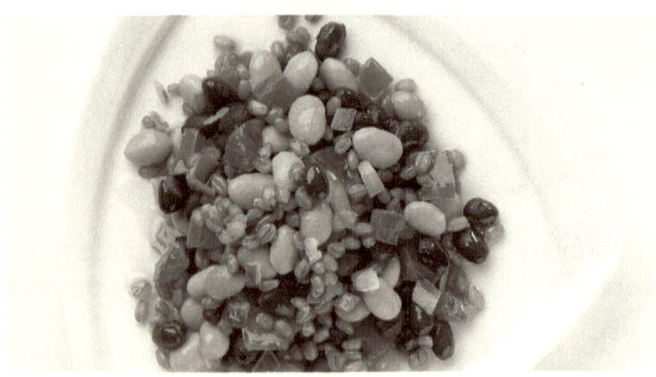

This recipe offers a delicious way to enjoy a salad with a difference. This is not something which can be made quickly, but the wait is well worth it.

Ingredients

- 4 cups water
- 1/2 cup dry wheat berries
- 1 cup black beans (cooked)
- 1 cup frozen (shelled edamame, thawed)
- 1 cup tomato (chopped)
- 1/2 cup red onion (finely chopped)
- 2 tbsp red wine vinegar
- 3 tbsp extra-virgin olive oil
- Salt and freshly ground pepper to taste

Method

1. Place the wheat berries in a saucepan, add the water, and bring to a boil. Then this should be covered, and left to simmer for approximately 55 minutes or until the wheat berries are tender.

2. Using a fine mesh strainer, the berries should be drained, and then mixed with all other ingredients.

3. It can be served immediately or refrigerated for up to 8 hours; if keeping chilled it should be covered with plastic to keep the salad fresh.

Top Fitness Tips of Today!

1. **Get Fit Not Skinny**- When you are dieting, and you are doing your workout plans. Get motivated about getting fit, not skinny. Your workouts should include flexibility, cardio, and strength.

2. **Do Not Eat White Things**- Most of the products today that are the white colors, should not be consumed when dieting. For example, things like white bread, flour, sugar, rice, and pasta should not be consumed. The only exemptions for white substances products include egg whites, cauliflower, and fish.

3. **Broccoli**- Broccoli is the best vegetable to choose when on a diet because it cleanses the liver.

4. **Vitamin D**- Getting the right amount of vitamin D is important because it aids in appetite. If you don't consume enough vitamin D, you can increase your appetite.

5. **Drink Water**- Drinking more water can aid in your weight loss journey. It keeps you energized.

6. **Tea**- Drinking tea and help you lose weight and feel better. Tea can help with your weight by increasing your metabolism.

Final Words

I would like to thank you for downloading my book and I hope I have been able to help you and educate you about something new.

If you have enjoyed this book and would like to share your positive thoughts, could you please take 30 seconds of your time to go back and give me a review on my Amazon book page!

I greatly appreciate seeing these reviews because it helps me share my hard work!

Again, thank you and I wish you all the best with your cooking journey!

Last Chance to Get YOUR Bonus!

FOR A LIMITED TIME ONLY – Get Olivia's best-selling book *"The #1 Cookbook: Over 170+ of the Most Popular Recipes Across 7 Different Cuisines!"* absolutely FREE!

Readers have absolutely loved this book because of the wide variety of recipes. It is highly recommended you check these recipes out and see what you can add to your home menu!

Once again, as a big thank-you for downloading this book, I'd like to offer it to you *100% FREE for a LIMITED TIME ONLY!*

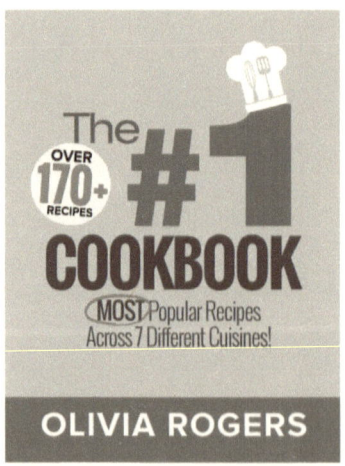

Get your free copy at:

TheMenuAtHome.com/Bonus

Disclaimer

This book and related site provides recipe and food advice in an informative and educational manner only, with information that is general in nature and that is not specific to you, the reader. The contents of this book and related site are intended to assist you and other readers in your personal efforts. Consult your physician or nutritionist regarding the applicability of any information provided in our information to you.

Nothing in this book should be construed as personal advice or diagnosis, and must not be used in this manner. The information provided about conditions is general in nature. This information does not cover all possible uses, actions, precautions, side-effects, or interactions of medicines, or medical procedures. The information in this site should not be considered as complete and does not cover all diseases, ailments, physical conditions, or their treatment.

No Warranties: The authors and publishers don't guarantee or warrant the quality, accuracy, completeness, timeliness, appropriateness or suitability of the information in this book, or of any product or services referenced by this site.

The information in this site is provided on an "as is" basis and the authors and publishers make no representations or warranties of any kind with respect to this information. This site may contain inaccuracies, typographical errors, or other errors.

Liability Disclaimer: The publishers, authors, and other parties involved in the creation, production, provision of information, or delivery of this site specifically disclaim any responsibility, and shall not be held liable for any damages, claims, injuries, losses, liabilities, costs, or obligations including any direct, indirect, special, incidental, or consequences damages (collectively known as "Damages") whatsoever and howsoever caused, arising out of, or in connection with the use or misuse of the site and the information contained within it, whether such Damages arise in contract, tort, negligence, equity, statute law, or by way of other legal theory.

www.ingramcontent.com/pod-product-compliance
Lightning Source LLC
Chambersburg PA
CBHW031126080526
44587CB00011B/1124